The Healthiest Kid
in the
Neighborhood

The Healthiest Kid
in the
Neighborhood

*Ten Ways to Get Your Family
on the Right Nutritional Track*

William Sears, M.D., Martha Sears, R.N.,
James Sears, M.D., and Robert Sears, M.D.

Little, Brown and Company
Boston New York London

Little, Brown and Company
Hachette Book Group USA
1271 Avenue of the Americas, New York, NY 10020
Visit our Web site at HachetteBookGroupUSA.com

First Edition: September 2006

Library of Congress Cataloging-in-Publication Data
The healthiest kid in the neighborhood : ten ways to get your family on the right nutritional track / William Sears . . . [et al.].
p. cm.
Includes index.
ISBN-10: 0-316-06012-7 (trade pbk.)
ISBN-13: 978-0-316-06012-7 (trade pbk.)
1. Children — Nutrition — Popular works.   2. Obesity in children — Prevention — Popular works.   3. Children — Health and hygiene — Popular works.
I. Sears, William, Dr.

RJ206.H34 2006
618.92'39 — dc22   2006002597

10   9   8   7   6   5   4   3   2   1

Q-MART

Designed by Bernard Klein
Drawings by Scott Herman

Printed in the United States of America

To our children — the healthiest kids in the neighborhood

James
Robert
Peter
Hayden
Erin
Matthew
Stephen
Lauren
—W.S. and M.S.

Leanne
Jonathan
— J.S.

Andrew
Alex
Joshua
— R.S.

Contents

4: Feed Your Family a Right-Fat Diet *91*

5: Feed Your Kids Grow Foods *116*

6: Raise a Grazer *146*

7: Eleven Ways to Feed Growing Brains *168*

8: Feed Your Family Immunity-Boosting Foods *194*

9: Raise a Lean Family *210*

VISIT DR. SEARS ONLINE

www.AskDrSears.com

Now you can access thousands of pages of nutritional, medical, and parenting information written by the Drs. Sears. Our comprehensive online resource expands on many of the topics discussed in *The Healthiest Kid in the Neighborhood.* We continuously update the information on our website to provide you with the latest on parenting and health-care issues. AskDrSears .com offers valuable insights on such topics as pregnancy and childbirth, infant feeding, family nutrition, discipline and behavior, fussy babies, and sleep problems. Our website also includes these unique features:

- The Food Forum, an interactive forum where parents share their favorite recipes and feeding strategies, and the Drs. Sears add their comments
- Downloadable Traffic-Light Eating chart
- *The Healthiest Kid in the Neighborhood* updates, updates of out-of-date information and discussions of new information about health and nutrition
- Additional recipes
- Our recommendations for the highest-quality and best-researched vitamins, minerals, omega 3's, and other nutritional supplements. We personally research all the supplements we recommend on our website, often going as far as visiting the manufacturer to see how the supplements are made. By going right to the source of the supplements, we can honestly say that these are the brands that we feel secure enough to give to our own families.
- Frequently Asked Questions answered
- Monthly newsletters
- Dr. Sears's Medicine Cabinet, a parent's guide to over-the-counter medications, including specific dose information

The Healthiest Kid
in the
Neighborhood

1

Getting on the Right Track:
Ten Nutritional Changes to Get Your
Child on a Healthy Path

Parents, we have a nutrition crisis in America. Children are feeding their growing bodies alarming amounts of junk food. Parents worry about the consequences. As pediatricians, we see the consequences. Junk-food diets are associated with serious health problems in childhood and in future adulthood. Consider these scary statistics:

- *Diabetes is on the rise.* The U.S. Centers for Disease Control, the government-funded research agency that tracks health trends in America, warns that unless American families change the way they eat and live, one in three children born in the year 2000 will develop diabetes. This is a sobering statistic. Diabetes can lead to heart disease, stroke, blindness, kidney failure, foot and leg amputations, pregnancy complications, and death related to influenza and pneumonia. Pediatricians predict that for the first time in American history, children will have a shorter, sicker lifespan than their parents have.

- *American kids are getting sicker.* When I (Bill) was in pediatric training, conditions such as Type 2 diabetes (high blood sugar) and cardiovascular disease (high cholesterol and high blood pressure) were known as adult-onset diseases. Since these conditions rarely appeared in children, pediatricians didn't need to learn much about them. Not so anymore. Doctors are seeing so many children with high blood sugar and high cholesterol levels that we no longer think of these conditions as beginning in adulthood. Even during the writing of this book, we saw kids with these "highs" along with other early signs of cardiovascular disease. In fact, in autopsy studies of children, fatty deposits have been found in the coronary arteries of children as young as one year of age. We know that these diseases are linked to certain ways of eating. It is indeed serious to see the effects appearing so early in life.

- *American kids are becoming sadder.* The number of children on mood-modifying drugs to perk them up or calm them down has increased drastically over the last ten years. Approximately 10 percent of school-age kids are now labeled as having A.D.D. (Attention Deficit Disorder) or various other types of learning disabilities. The reasons for this are many. As you will learn in chapter 7, Eleven Ways to Feed Growing Brains, the brain is the organ most affected (for better or worse) by nutrition.

- *American kids are getting fatter.* The surgeon general of the United States now ranks excess weight and obesity as the number-one public-health concern. The disease consequences of obesity are greater than those of any infectious disease. Obesity-related illnesses kill almost as many Americans each year as tobacco. You warn your children about the health risks of smoking. Being overweight carries similar risks.

What's the cause of this health crisis? Food, glorious food! In America, food — or the abuse of it — is making kids sick. Over and over again, research reveals that poor eating habits put adults at risk for serious illnesses including diabetes, cardiovascular disease, some cancers (including breast and colon cancer), and the "-itis" illnesses (e.g., arthritis, colitis, bronchitis). Eating habits are formed in childhood. Children who eat healthily are much more likely to be healthy, both as children and as adults. Kids who live on junk food are more likely to get sick and to become victims of these diseases in adulthood — if not sooner. It's as straightforward as that.

Hippocrates once said, "Let food be your medicine." The ancient physician was right. Good food keeps people well. We eat food for three reasons: for growth, for pleasure, and for "medicine." While most processed foods get a passing grade for being pleasurable and providing energy, most make a failing grade for their medicinal or health-promoting properties. In a nutshell, that's the most important difference between real, wholesome fresh foods and processed ones.

Our bodies function best when they are well nourished. We want you to value food not only for the pleasure it brings and the energy it provides but also for its ability to keep your body functioning at its very best. That's the theme of this book — how choosing the right foods can make your children (and you) healthier. The sicker, sadder, fatter picture described above is not inevitable. By following the advice and making the changes we suggest in this book, your children can be the healthiest kids in the neighborhood.

THE FOOD-HEALTH CONNECTION: DR. BILL'S STORY

During my thirty-five years as a pediatrician, I've learned a lot by studying my patients. I think of my office as a sort of research laboratory, where I can look for connections between what children and parents do in the early years of life and what happens when these kids become teens and adults.

I conducted studies in my "laboratory." My first "study group" was composed of the children of parents (usually moms) whom

I dubbed "pure moms" — those who never let a morsel of junk food pollute their children's growing bodies. In my less-informed years, I referred to them as "health-food nuts." As I followed these "pure children" of "pure parents" through childhood and adolescence, I noticed that these kids were not sick as often as most children. And when they did get sick, their illnesses were less severe, and they recovered sooner. These "pure" kids had fewer of the usual childhood illnesses such as ear infections, colds, and intestinal upsets, and usually they recovered from these illnesses with little or no help from me.

I also noticed that these kids had healthier brains. When they entered school, they were less likely to be tagged with such labels as A.D.D. or learning disabled. Rarely was I called upon to prescribe behavior- or mood-altering medications for these "pure" kids. I eventually grew convinced that these kids were biochemically better off because of what their parents fed them. What was going on inside these kids at the cellular or even molecular level? I wondered. (On page 29 you will learn how "pure" kids are biochemically and molecularly better off.) Initially I dismissed as just a curiosity the connection between food and health that I observed. And then the subject became personal.

Cancer caused me to care. Even though I was beginning to see the connection between food and mental and physical health, I was not yet motivated to change my own eating habits, much less to write a book about nutrition and health. It wasn't something I could get excited about, because I hadn't yet experienced the food-health connection personally. Then in April of 1997 I was diagnosed with colon cancer — and not just early-stage colon cancer, but the kind serious enough to threaten my life. I had surgery and underwent both chemotherapy and radiation. It was a very difficult time for me, for Martha, and for our entire family, and I vowed that I would do whatever it took to help my body fight the cancer and to prevent its return.

As I learned more about colon cancer, I had to acknowledge that my lifestyle had put me at risk. A lack of physical activity and a low-fiber, high-fat diet are known risk factors for colon cancer, along with obesity, alcohol consumption, and tobacco use. I didn't smoke or abuse alcohol, nor was I much overweight, but I had to confess that my eating habits were far from ideal, and they had been that way since my childhood. While fighting the cancer, I made big changes in my lifestyle to prevent its return. If I hadn't made the changes described in this chapter, I might not have lived to write this book.

Nutrition became my mission. Getting parents and children excited about good nutrition has become part of my mission in life. After my battle with cancer, I wanted every family in our pediatric practice to be a "pure family." Soon, every well-child visit included a minicourse, or even a loving lecture, on what parents should feed their kids. I shared what I had learned about healthy eating with all my patients, because my studies had shown me that the same nutritional program that cures old colons grows healthy kids.

In this book, we will describe ten nutritional changes that every family can make — *must* make — to help their kids live longer and healthier lives. What a difference I've noticed in myself, my family, and our young patients when these changes are made!

How to Get Started

When I began my own eating program, I had two powerful motivators: love and fear. I loved my family and feared the return of cancer. Certainly these motivating factors were enough to get me started. Many people start diets, plans, and programs with equally strong motivation. Yet it's hard to change old habits, even when there are good reasons for doing so. What made it possible for me to stick with the program? Here are a few tips.

Become obsessed! In order to change your body or your child's body, you first have to change your mind. Early on in my new eating program, I realized that change doesn't come easily. During the first few months, I felt a strong urge to let go and settle back into my old lifestyle. Yet my motivation to change was also strong. The result of this conflict? I became obsessed with good eating. I knew that the first few months of a lifestyle change are the hardest part for most people, because the new way of doing things has not yet become part of how they live. To counteract that all-too-human resistance to change, I put all of my energy into being fanatical about health and well-being. For a while, nutrition books and scientific journals were all over the house, and not one, but two juicers took up space on our kitchen counter. I feel that this initial obsession was like my way of paying my dues before being admitted into the lifelong club of healthier living.

Make a project out of your problem. As I began my "I don't want to get cancer again" program, I became interested in the specific health strategies of people who have survived major illnesses or tragedies and gone on to live healthier and richer lives. What I learned was that survivors make a project out of their problem. They study their problem. They find the best resources available and learn from them. As much as possible, they take control of their problem. Together with their health-care providers, they participate in decisions about what changes they need to make. So this is what I did, too — I turned my problem into a project, into an opportunity to learn and to change. You can do this as well. Take your concerns about your family's health and your children's future and turn them into a serious project. This will help you make healthy changes in your family's eating habits and lifestyle.

Show me the science. I realized I had to get smart before I could get healthy. I'd be more likely to stick with a nutritional change if I knew the reason for making it. So I became a student again. I read hundreds of books and articles on health and nutrition, and I found that many fascinating nutrition studies lie buried in obscure medical journals that are read only by university professors. The results of these studies get little public attention, and if they do, they are often contradicted by other results, leaving the public wondering what to believe. I quickly realized that I had to separate fact from fiction and make judgments about which studies were credible and important and which ones were less conclusive or perhaps even wrong. As a doctor, I am trained to think critically and to base the advice I give my patients on strong scientific evidence. So "show me the science" became my motto — for my own lifestyle changes and for the eating plan suggested in this book. Because few parents are able to be so discerning about nutritional science, throughout this book I've done it for you. My life depended on accurate nutritional information, and so does the health of your children.

In search of the perfect diet, I quickly learned that few of the popular diet books are based on sound science, and most are nothing more than quick-fix fads whose popularity fades when the next diet fad comes along. I wanted a diet that stood up to scientific scrutiny and that I could follow for the rest of my life. Besides, weight loss was not my main goal; lean and healthy was my goal. It made no sense to be at an optimal weight without enjoying optimal health. And eating is supposed to be pleasurable. Most diets fail because they take much of the pleasure out of eating. Who wants to spend so much time counting carbs, fat grams, or calories only to wind up feeling deprived? I wanted an eating plan that was healthy and that I would enjoy following.

Better Ways to Eat

My quest for scientific information on healthy eating styles led me to population studies — research on correlations between the eating habits and the health of certain groups of people who share a culture and an eating style. I believe that population studies are some of the most meaningful, because they study a lot of people over a long time, not just for months or years, but for decades.

So what was my new diet going to be? When I began my quest for the perfect way to eat, the low-carb craze was regaining popularity. But I knew from population studies that Asians eat a relatively high-carbohydrate diet — and they are some of the leanest and healthiest people in the world. Unlike in the typical American diet, however, with its heavy emphasis on processed, packaged foods, the carbs in the Asian diet come mainly from fresh vegetables, grains, and legumes. It seemed that low-carb wasn't the answer. I needed a right-carb diet.

What about a low-fat diet? Population studies show also that some of the healthiest people in the world and with the lowest incidence of heart disease, such as Eskimos and people of the Mediterranean, don't eat a low-fat diet. The fatty foods they eat are high in certain kinds of fatty acids, especially the group known as omega-3 fats. Again, I found myself rejecting the concept of a low-fat diet in favor of a right-fat diet.

Besides a right-carb and right-fat diet, what about protein? I discovered a curious quirk about protein. It's not just for muscle builders. Of all the nutrients, protein satisfies the appetite most quickly and with less than half the calories of fat. And it's very hard to overeat protein. My healthy diet would have to include enough protein.

*   *   *

My eating habits have rubbed off on my kids. Dr. Bob shares his experience:

My wife and I were sitting in our living room the night before Easter, filling our kids' baskets with candy and chocolate in every form possible. It suddenly dawned on me: I'm going to eat about ten pieces of chocolate tonight and several pieces each day for the next two months (the kids never seemed to notice that their Easter treats disappeared faster than they were eating them). It shocked me. I was already getting a stomachache from just the thought of it. Then I wondered, Do I have the willpower to just say no for this Easter season and to go off all candy and sugary food? I went for it, and now I don't even put sugar in my coffee anymore. The only vice I allow myself is homemade desserts. Two years later, I'm 15 pounds lighter, feel great, and am still candy free. It's amazing how much my mom's healthy eating rules have influenced me. All those years as a kid without junk food in the house seem to have paid off.

The population studies I read, along with other scientific information about specific kinds of fats and carbohydrates, helped me understand what nutrients my body needed to stay healthy. But we don't buy, prepare, and eat nutrients; we eat food. It was up to me to turn the information about good nutrition into a healthy eating plan. This was where the fun began. As I sought out the nutrition that would help me stay healthy, I gained a new appreciation for all kinds of good food — fresh fish, brightly colored fruits and vegetables, and a variety of whole grains. I changed the way I ate by seeking out the foods that contained the important nutrients my body needed. Over the years, as I have shared this eating style with family members, friends, and patients, it has evolved into the eating action plan that we outline in the chapters of this book.

TEN CHANGES EVERY FAMILY MUST MAKE

Our eating plan for healthy kids and parents is summarized in the ten changes listed below — changes we believe every family must make in order to raise healthy kids. We will show you more science about this eating plan in the chapters ahead. (Look for the boxes headed "Science Says.") For now, here's a summary of what we have learned about the healthiest way to eat. Making these changes will keep your child from becoming one of those unhealthy statistics you read about at the beginning of this chapter.

1. Shape young tastes *early*.
2. Feed your family the *right carbs*.
3. Feed your family the *right fats*.
4. Feed your children *grow foods*.
5. Feed your family *fill-up foods*.
6. Begin the day with a *brainy breakfast*.
7. Raise a *grazer*.
8. Feed your child's *immune system*.
9. Raise a *lean* family. Get active as a family.
10. Teach your children to be wise supermarket *shoppers*.

Is this just another diet plan? Yes and no. Yes, if you understand the word "diet" in its original meaning in Greek: a way of living. No, if your concept of diet implies deprivation. A diet that is mostly "don't eat this" and "don't eat that" will be hard to start and even harder to stick to. In the chapters ahead, we will accentuate the positive — all the good foods your family will enjoy with this new way of eating.

THE RESULTS: A HEALTHIER SEARS FAMILY, A HEALTHIER PEDIATRIC PRACTICE

Within a few months of following this new eating program, I (Bill) noticed big changes, literally from head to toe. I had more energy, craved healthy foods, shunned processed stuff, and generally felt better than I had in my whole life. Because I had personally experienced the connection between eating well and feeling well, I eventually got our whole family, including sons Jim and Bob and their families, to a whole new level of awareness. Jim and Bob began to experience the same wonderful results, so I then had two partners who were also passionate. Now all three of us share our program with the families in our medical practice. Here are the changes that parents report in their kids:

Healthier food cravings. When I was six weeks into my new eating program, I noticed that I was beginning to crave the things that made me feel better. I still had a sweet tooth, yet I preferred to satisfy it with the good carbs in fresh fruit, with the occasional bit of dark chocolate, rather than with the junk carbs in cakes and cookies. I craved seafood and veggies and ate only whole-grain bread and pasta. In the early stages of my new eating plan, my mind had to dictate to my body what to eat. But after my body began to get the nutrients it needed, it started to ask for more of the good stuff. There is evidence that food cravings have a biochemical basis, and, indeed, something about my biology had changed. After several months of eating healthier food, my body started reminding me, "Gotta have it!" It kept me on the right track.

The same thing happens now in our practice. Parents frequently report, "Now he seems to want to eat healthy food like vegetables. Before, I couldn't get them into him." Their children started asking for seafood and veggies and ate less bread and pasta. As we mentioned above, this makes biochemical sense. This is called metabolic programming, which you will learn about later.

HOLIDAY GUT FEELINGS

At first holidays were a challenge for me. All the traditions about festive food tempted me to revert back to my precancer diet. But I quickly realized I had developed what I call AFI — artificial food intolerance. A glass of corn syrup–sweetened eggnog left me feeling yucky. The "brain" in my gut seemed to be telling me, "Don't go there. Don't drink that stuff again." That "stuff" never used to bother me, but it should have. The list of ingredients on the eggnog carton read like a chemical formula!

Our eating program will *change your kids' cravings!* Those four magic words will make this style of eating work for your family. Many makeover programs don't go far enough to bring about lasting change in a person's basic biochemistry. The great thing about our program is that once you get to a certain point, your body craves whatever it needs in order to stay there. You'll find that even if you crave a cookie, you want a healthier cookie — and just one! (You can read more about changing children's cravings on page 40.)

More stamina. Parents in our practice tell us that they notice this change in their children, and so did I in myself. Three months into my program, I noticed that my resting heart rate and breathing rate were lower. My body was now acting like an engine that was tuned up and energy efficient. We took up swing dancing as a couple hobby. Martha called me "Zip."

Better brains. I experienced a lot of mental perks from the program as well. I noticed fewer mood swings, and I managed my feelings better. I was more consistently upbeat and handled stress better. My brain was more focused. What's good for the body is also good for the brain. When children eat the right foods, their parents and teachers notice an improvement in their school performance. These children are able to focus better, and they have fewer behavioral and attention problems at school and at home. In fact, in children, the behavioral effects of better nutrition are even more noticeable than the physical changes.

More acute senses. At a baseball game one evening, I realized I had forgotten my glasses, which I needed in order to see the outfield scoreboard. But when I looked up, I was surprised that for the first time in ten years, I could read the scoreboard without glasses. Also, my sense of smell became more acute and discerning. Smelly substances in the air bothered me more. I began to go out of my way to avoid driving behind buses and trucks with their exhaust fumes.

Healthier skin and gums. For years in our pediatric practice I have noticed that infants and children with healthy diets have healthier skin. Children who eat more fruits, vegetables, and omega-3 fats have skin that is less dry and flaky, especially during the low-humidity winter months. Cuts and scratches heal faster, and eczema is rarely a problem. Also, for many years I had had severe gum problems (gingivitis). After I'd been on my new eating plan for several months, my dentist noticed a difference and remarked, "Your gums look great! What are you doing differently?"

Ah, that good gut feeling! The most striking change I noticed was a good feeling inside my gut. Our young patients experience the same effect when, as they report, they stop eating foods that give them "yuck tummy." That new good feeling helped motivate me to stick with my eating program. A voice deep in my gastrointestinal system cried, "No!" whenever I contemplated eating an unhealthful food.

That voice really does come from the gut. The lining and muscular wall of the intestines are richly supplied with nerves. In fact, there are more nerves in the intestines than in the spinal cord. These nerves send messages to your child's brain about whether his gut feels good or bad after he eats a certain food. The next time he thinks about eating that same food, those nerve pathways and stored memories light up, and both the head brain and the gut brain remember whether it is a healthy food. At least it's supposed to work that way. After years of unhealthy eating, the gut brain shuts down because it hasn't been listened to.

Another benefit of our program is that your stomach will never feel too full or too empty. This is because you'll eat often, in small amounts — a pattern we call "grazing." You won't feel hungry, so you won't feel deprived, and your gut brain will never feel uncomfortably full either.

Two "pure parents" recently shared this story with me (Dr. Bill) during their child's five-year checkup: "When he drinks one of those junk drinks at school, the ones with a lot of coloring, he turns into somebody we don't even know." I asked the child how these drinks made him feel. He replied, "My tummy feels awful." After congratulating the family on shaping their child's tastes in the right direction, I explained to them what was going on inside their child's body. His body, especially his central nervous system, was so used to the metabolic effects of real food that when the artificial stuff entered his system, some internal sensor said, in effect, "Whoa! This stuff doesn't belong here." The huge network of nerves that line the gut had been so programmed to experience the effects of real foods that they rebelled at the gut feel of junk food. These parents not only shaped their child's taste, they programmed his "gut feelings."

Upgrading to finer dining. Within six months of changing your family's way of eating, your children will become picky eaters — in a good way. They will be more discriminating about the quality of the food they put into their gut. Fruits and vegetables will need to be fresh or frozen, not canned. They may stay away from processed foods, which can be far too salty for their sensitive taste buds. Sauces will need to be lighter and less greasy. Seafood will have to be baked or grilled, not fried. Salad greens will have to be green, not pale. Bread will have to be whole grain, not white. Their bodies will demand quality food. This will be the beginning, not the end, of fine dining.

In my precancer years I enjoyed spicy foods only occasionally. Why now did I find myself often craving chili peppers and dishes heavily seasoned with curry, turmeric, and garlic? My research unearthed some predictable answers: The body, in its wisdom, knows these spicy foods are full of phytonutrients, natural anti-cancer, anti-aging, and anti-inflammatory substances. I even began to enjoy eating tofu, a food I once made fun of. And the blood-sugar-stabilizing effect of cinnamon explains why I started putting a hefty dose of it in my daily smoothie.

Of course, I got the expected protests from our children. One day, eight-year-old Lauren said, "Daddy, I liked it better before you got cancer. Our food wasn't so weird, and we got more junk food."

THE RIGHT TRACK

Our eating program is not a diet in the usual sense, with the goal of losing a certain number of pounds or lowering blood cholesterol to a certain level. Instead, it's an eating program (remember the meaning of the word "diet" in Greek is "a way of living") for optimal performance and optimal health. It's about not weight loss but health gain. It's all about thriving. "Thrive" is a word we have used in many of our parenting books to describe optimal development: children becoming the best they can be — mentally, physically, and emotionally. Thriving is also the goal of this eating program. It's not just about avoiding the dangers of obesity, high blood pressure, diabetes, and other nutrition-related diseases. It's about a lifetime of wellness for both the body and the brain.

The ten steps that we have taken in our families can instill in your children healthy habits for life. There is scientific evidence that eating and exercise habits formed in childhood program not only the mind for good habits in adulthood but also the body. This relatively new concept among nutrition researchers is called metabolic programming, and this is what goes on inside the "pure kids" we observe in our pediatric practice. Their mothers' early vigilance about what they are eating shapes their tastes and sets up their bodies' metabolic programming, so they naturally choose the foods that are good for them. This long-term benefit — the lasting effects of metabolic programming — may be the most important reason for changing your family's eating and activity patterns now. Now, as part of routine pediatric checkups, we explain the importance of healthy metabolic programming to parents. One mother later proudly told us, "I'm a metabolically minded mother."

As you will learn in chapter 2, metabolic programming gets your children on the right nutritional track at the cellular level. They become so biochemically balanced that they feel well when they stay on track and unwell if they get off track. These early good nutritional habits will become so imprinted on their sense of well-being that they are likely to hang on to them for life.

How to Get Started

If your family's eating habits are way off the right track, they will want to know what's going on when suddenly there are cases of bottled water instead of soda in the pantry and fruit instead of cookies in their lunch boxes. Here's how to get children — and reluctant parents (usually dads) — to change their attitudes about eating well.

Just do it! The first step in making any change in lifestyle is believing that it matters. Let your family sense your passion and your convictions about healthy eating. Your children get their values from you. Younger children accept their parents' convictions without question, and even older children and teenagers are influenced by what their parents believe and do, in addition to messages from peers, teachers, and the media.

Make it a family value. Tell and show your family, "This is how we eat." Your children will be most receptive if you start early, before their young tastes have been shaped in the wrong direction. Yet anytime before age six or seven, kids will follow what we call the "we principle" — how *we* do things in *our* family. The idea that "we eat healthy food in our family" can be contagious, a sort of infectious wellness that spreads throughout the whole family. Let everyone know that the "new" way of eating is not just the result of mom reading another book or dad being told by the doctor that his cholesterol is a little high. It's a permanent change. Make healthy eating a family value, a natural part of your family's life, just as you share other important values with your children, such as, "We don't *talk* like that in our family. We don't *act* like that. *This* is what we believe, *this* is how we behave, and *this* is what we eat." It's as simple as that!

"INSTEAD OF . . . TRY . . ."

To shape your child's tastes toward healthier choices, carry around a mental "instead of . . ." list such as this one:

Instead of . . .	Try . . .
soda	part sparkling water, part 100 percent fruit juice
juice drinks	part 100 percent juice, part water
sweeteners in cereal (sugar, corn syrup) or syrup on pancakes	blueberries, cinnamon, fruit toppings
candy bars	fruit, yogurt, nuts
ice cream	gelato (see recipe, page 319)
french fries	sweet potato fries (at home); fruit or guacamole (eating out)
butter on bread	dipping bread in olive oil
white bread	100 percent whole grain
beef burger	veggie burger, fish taco, salmon patty
salad dressing	hummus, olive oil and vinegar, lemon juice
"enriched" wheat pasta	whole-grain pasta
sour cream	plain full-fat yogurt
mashed potatoes and gravy	broccoli and homemade cheese sauce

Show your care and concern. Let your children know that you care about what they eat because you care about them. "Because we love you and want you to be healthy, we can't let you pollute your body . . ." Kids may protest at first and tell you that they want junk food and that it's not fair that they can't eat the foods their friends do. Yet down deep they will sense you are right. It may take a while, but eventually they will get it. Someday you will hear them say to a friend, "I don't eat that stuff anymore."

Educate them. Kids deserve to know why you're serving veggies and peanut butter sandwiches instead of chicken nuggets and french fries for lunch. So tell them! "This food will help you grow, that food is bad for your body." When your children hear about good food, eat good food, and live a healthy lifestyle day after day, they will come to appreciate the important role that nutrition plays in good health.

THE HIGHER COST OF HEALTH

"But fresh and organic food costs more!" you may protest. "What's your child's health worth?" we reply. Oftentimes in our office we see a financially pinched parent holding a $4 cup of coffee while her child is munching on a bag of junk chips. You'll save a lot of money on medical bills and missed workdays by spending money on real food. Consider it part of your health-insurance budget and a wise long-term investment.

Become a spin doctor. Be sure your children don't regard these changes in your family's way of eating as deprivation. Remind them that eating healthy food and taking good care of their bodies is far more important than the instant gratification they might get from a Twinkie or a bag of Doritos. Put a positive spin on the differences they may perceive between how their family eats and how their friends' families eat. Remember, it's all in the presentation. You might even want to drop the term "healthy food," which some kids equate with "icky." We have found that children enjoy a lighthearted approach to nutrition, so we use fun terms, such as "grow foods," "sick foods," "feel-better foods," and "red-light" and "green-light foods." These are terms you will read throughout this book. Also, relate healthy eating with looks and performance, using such terms as "pretty-hair foods" or "run-faster foods."

How Your Children Might React

Initially, you may experience resistance from your children as you serve them new foods and banish junk food from your house. That's to be expected. Children, just like adults, resist change, and it's harder for some to change than for others. Some kids feel only the immediate loss — no more take-out cheeseburgers for dinner — and don't see the long-term health benefits. Once it sinks in that this new way of eating is here to stay, they will accept it, even if they are not enthusiastic about it. ("I guess this is the way we're going to eat from now on. I might as well get used to it. I miss going to McDonald's, but that's just the way my parents are . . .")

After a few months of better eating and more exercise, your children will notice a difference in how they feel. They will discover that they can run faster and longer. They won't tire out in the middle of a soccer game, and they'll have the energy for long bike rides. They will enjoy being active, because inside it makes them feel calm, happy, and right. They will be more alert in school and better able to concentrate. They may not know how to describe all these good feelings, but they will know something good is happening in their bodies — and in their brains. Help them to understand that these good results are directly related to the good food they eat.

IT'S OKAY TO BE A 90/10 FAMILY

Eating is supposed to be pleasurable; otherwise the human race would not have survived. That's an important message to keep in mind in feeding your family. Coming on as too restrictive is likely to backfire, causing your children to sneak sweet treats at friends' homes or trade lunches at school. Even many of the "pure parents" in our practice reveal that it helps to be what they call a "90/10" family — eating very healthy food 90 percent of the time once the kids are old enough to be influenced by other eating styles. For many kids, even being an 80/20 family would be a marked improvement. In fact, you're likely to notice that once you get your children on the right track, they may "need" an occasional sweet treat, but they won't overdose on them. We've noticed that when our children have an occasional stop at a fast-food joint with friends, it serves as a reminder that junk food makes them feel junky inside afterward. That's the beauty of being on the right track. Once your children get on it, they will naturally shun overdosing on, or even indulging in, junk food because of the junky feelings they get when they do. Now our kids would scold *us* if we were to stop at a hamburger joint.

Kids monitoring parents. After a few months of following this healthier way of eating, parents often tell us, "When my children catch me eating junk food, they advise me, 'Mom, that's a red-light food,' or 'That's not a grow food.' I like that."

The final stage in changing your children's way of eating comes when they begin to prefer the good food and choose it when they are away from home. Your way of eating becomes their way of eating. They will select a salad over a cheeseburger and fill up on veggies rather than potato chips at parties. The occasional junk-food lapse is no longer perceived as a treat, because your child recognizes the yucky feelings that follow and attributes them to the unhealthy food. When your children reach this point, you've got them! They are hooked on good eating. Their metabolism is programmed to prefer healthy food. The internal wisdom of the body will let them know if they get off the right track, and they will recognize that the tiredness and the mental fog weren't worth that second or larger piece of gooey birthday cake. A healthy way of eating will be a part of your child for the rest of his life.

WHY PARENTS AREN'T SO "PURE"

One day while standing at the checkout counter at a local supermarket, I (Bill) noticed the mother in front of me unloading her shopping cart piled high with junk food: fiberless cereals, sweetened beverages, packaged lunches, gelatin desserts, and "bakery bads." I wondered if she had simply forgotten to shop the perimeter of the supermarket. Why would any mother feed this junk to her kids? I thought. Either she doesn't know it's junk or she doesn't care, which is not likely to be true. As a parent and pediatrician, I have tried to figure out why parents like this everyday shopper let their kids eat junk. Good food is readily available in America, and the parents I am talking about have enough money to buy it. So why do they buy it? The answer came to me as I was sitting in the boardroom of a major food-processing company a few years ago. Here's what I saw.

The problem. During the writing of this book, I was invited to spend a day consulting with executives of one of the leading producers of packaged foods. This company was genuinely exploring ways to market more nutritious foods to parents and kids in an effort to do something about the epidemic of obesity, diabetes, and other nutrition-related diseases among children. One of the executives opened the meeting with a statement about the food industry's dilemma: "We know we need to improve the nutritional quality of our food, but we hesitate to invest in the development and marketing of more nutritious foods. We're afraid that kids won't eat the food and parents won't buy it."

The marketing manager explained the product-development process: "Before the company launches a new packaged food, we taste-test the food on hundreds of children." The director of advertising added, "Of course, we have to make the package attractive so that kids perceive it as fun."

I asked about the food itself. "Your processed stuff is not whole food. What would happen if you made your packaged pastas from whole wheat instead of processed white flour?" The executives were quick to respond. "We tried that, and the kids wouldn't eat it." "What about yogurt?" I asked. "Why do you need to add so many sweeteners and food colorings to a healthy food like yogurt?" "We tested that," they responded, "but we found that kids prefer the sweetened, colored varieties."

As I picked up one of their competitors' packaged lunches from the table in front of me, I probed further. "The ingredient list reads like a chemistry set. This package should have a warning label on it: 'Hazardous to your child's health.' Why would parents buy such stuff?"

The response. The marketing director explained: "The main reasons why mothers buy packaged foods are that they're convenient and they know their children will eat them without a hassle. When we surveyed our buyers, mostly mothers, they admitted they were willing to sacrifice nutritional value for not having to hassle with their children about eating the food. The mothers suppressed their guilt over serving junk mac and cheese in return for not getting into fights with their kids."

I now had an explanation for why parents let their kids eat junk: Many parents are nutritional wimps. They are willing to sacrifice nutrition and health for convenience and the ease of feeding their kids foods they know they will eat. As a parent of eight children, I can sympathize. Modern parents are busy all day at work and at home. When dinnertime arrives, they want something they can serve

NUTSHELL

Here's the problem: Kids have lost their taste for real, wholesome food.

quickly that the kids are sure to eat. No muss, no fuss! Unfortunately, this means that kids, parents, and food sellers are caught in a vicious cycle. Parents know that they ought to serve their children nutritious food, but their kids have come to prefer highly processed, heavily advertised junk food. Food manufacturers cater to the market, reinforcing kids' tastes and parents' desire for convenience.

The solution. After my meeting with the product developers, I had a better understanding of what has to change if we are going to raise healthier kids who eat healthier food. First, parents need to understand that what they feed their kids matters. Parents instinctively want the best for their children in every aspect of life — the best school, the best manners, the best friends, and emotional and spiritual wholeness. They realize that these things are important to ensure happiness and success in life. Yet parents don't apply the same high standard to what their children eat. I believe that many parents simply do not know, or are not convinced, that junk food builds junk bodies and brains. All the confusing messages about food in the media and at the supermarket have led them to believe that what their children eat doesn't make much of a difference. Kids grow no matter what you feed them. To most parents, the health consequences of the typical American diet they share with their kids are too far in the future to make a difference in what they eat today. Parents need to be educated that feeding kids real, wholesome food will make them healthier for years to come.

Something else needs to change as well: children's tastes. Change has to start in the kitchens of American homes. It's up to parents to reshape their children's tastes. American children start out eating junk food so early that they believe processed food is what food is supposed to taste like. This is why the kids resist when Mom starts serving fresh, unprocessed foods. Yet it is possible to shape young tastes so that kids prefer the healthy foods that are good for them.

It's easy to blame the food industry when kids choose french fries, chicken nuggets, sugary cereals, and soda pop over fresh fruits and vegetables. But food companies are only responding to the demands of the marketplace. They sell what parents will buy and what kids will eat. That part of the situation is not going to change. It's up to parents to say no to junk food.

Dr. Bob shares a conversation he frequently has with parents:

Parents often complain to me, "All my kid eats is crackers, chips, cookies, and soda." My response to that is "So let me get this straight. Your child has a job, earns money, drives himself to the store, buys this food, and brings it home and eats it?" The parents' response is always the same. "Well, no. I buy it. My husband likes it, and I do, too." For some reason, the familiar quote from the movie Field of Dreams *always comes to mind at this point: "If you build it, they will come." Only here it's "If you buy it, they will eat it!"*

Kids can't eat junk food if parents don't buy it, and if parents stopped buying processed convenience foods, the food industry would have to change its ways and upgrade the stuff they put in those cute packages. In the next chapter you will hear what we would say if we had the opportunity to deliver a supermarket sermon to the mother with the cart full of junk food.

2

Shaping Young Tastes

Shaping young tastes is the key to improving your family's nutrition, and that's what you'll learn about in this chapter. We'll explain how shaping your child's tastes to prefer fresh, minimally processed foods will not only make your child healthier now but also program your child's body to stay healthy.

METABOLIC PROGRAMMING: THE KEY TO HEALTH

Parents know that key events in childhood can affect their child's personality and behavior as an adult. These events imprint themselves on children's minds and hearts and affect the way they react to situations later in life. Nutrition researchers believe that a similar kind of imprinting takes place in the body, a process called metabolic programming, which is the scientific basis for grandmother's wisdom "You are what you eat."

Metabolic programming, a concept we introduced in chapter 1, creates the *cellular blueprint* that determines how cells do their jobs. What children eat affects their metabolic programming. Cells that are programmed in the right way will be more resistant to disease in adulthood. In studying the "pure kids" in our practice, we have become convinced that these kids are biochemically better off at the cellular level. Here's how metabolic programming influences children's growth, development, and lifelong health.

Cells that eat better grow better. Your child's vital organs, such as the brain, the heart, and the liver, are only as healthy as the cells they are made of. Cells grow and divide rapidly during infancy and childhood. An excess or deficiency of certain nutrients at critical periods of growth may affect how well cells reproduce, how healthy these cells are, and how efficiently they work. Ultimately, how the cells work determines how well the organ works and how well the body functions, now and in the future.

Experiments have shown that metabolic programming is particularly important in liver cells. Young animals who get too much of some nutrients and not enough of others grow up to have defects in their liver cells. The liver plays an important role in the body's metabolism and growth, so there is reason to be concerned about defective liver cells. In one experiment, malnourished infant animals showed less growth of the insulin-secreting cells of the pancreas, a defect that could predispose them to diabetes as adults.

Metabolic programming seems to be especially important to brain cell development. Studies show that malnutrition during critical periods of brain growth can result in permanent deficits in brain function. There seems to be a window of opportunity for brain growth, a time when feeding practices have the most influence on long-term health and intelligence. This window of opportunity is open widest at the time when cells are growing and dividing the fastest — in infancy and early childhood. Imagine saying to the supermarket shopper with the cart full of junk, "Why would you feed your children such *dumb* foods?"

Genes that are fed better reproduce better. Cell reproduction follows the directions encoded in the cell's genes. A healthy diet stabilizes the strands of DNA that make up the genes, so the cells reproduce the way they're supposed to. A junk-food diet can make the DNA less stable, leading to faulty cell reproduction. Cells that don't reproduce exactly as they are supposed to may become cancer cells, or they may simply be unable to do their job well, making the child more susceptible to serious illnesses in later childhood and adulthood. Faulty genetic programming may be responsible for the four main groups of illnesses: degenerative diseases of the central nervous system; such as multiple sclerosis; metabolic problems such as diabetes; cardiovascular disorders; and inflammatory, or "-itis," illnesses. Consider the feeding practices you will learn in this book as your child's first visit to a neurologist, endocrinologist, cardiologist, and allergist. These "doctors" set up practice in your kitchen.

Don't worry that one junk-food binge will permanently affect your child's health. The effects of good or bad nutrition are dose related. A single serving of soda is unlikely to be harmful, but a can a day for a number of years is likely to damage cells throughout the body.

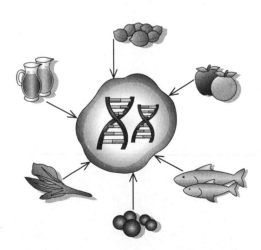

SCIENCE SAYS: EARLY FEEDING AFFECTS LATER HEALTH

Metabolic-programming research is in its infancy, but science has already found some connections between nutrition in early childhood and adult health.

- Experimental animals that were overfed with a high-carb junk-food diet as juveniles showed elevations in blood insulin and cholesterol levels when they were older. As adults, they had insulin-resistant Type 2 diabetes, due to a defect in insulin binding to the receptor sites on liver cell membranes. In other words, early nutrition affected the structure of the receptor sites on the surface of the cell, which in turn affected the cell's ability to recognize and regulate insulin.

- Experimental animals that were fed a diet high in saturated fats as juveniles grew up to have abnormal cholesterol metabolism, lower levels of protective, or good, cholesterol, HDL, and higher levels of the bad, or heart-damaging, cholesterol, LDL.

- Experimental animals that were overfed as juveniles had a higher incidence of insulin insensitivity, or Type 2 diabetes, as adults.

- In his book *Health and Nutrition Secrets That Can Change Your Life,* neurosurgeon Russell Blaylock reports that young animals that were fed flavor enhancers such as MSG showed microscopic changes in the brain and grew up to exhibit autistic-like behaviors, in addition to preferring high-carb foods and becoming obese.

Cells that eat better function better in the body. Genes all by themselves do not determine whether a person will be healthy or not. The body is more complicated than that. Many factors affect how genes are expressed — that is, what effect they have on the body. One of the newest and most promising fields of research is called nutrigenomics (science jargon for "we are what we eat"), the study of how nutrition affects our genes. In an individual who is genetically prone to a certain disease, nutrition may influence the expression of whatever genes are linked to that disease. For example, a person with a genetic predisposition to Type 2 diabetes is more likely to become diabetic if he or she eats a diet high in junk carbs. Someone without the Type 2 diabetes gene is less likely to be affected by a poor diet. Another example: Researchers have found a genetic quirk called the angiotensin gene (angiotensin is one of the body's blood pressure–regulating hormones). People who have this gene are more likely to develop high blood pressure when they eat excessive amounts of salt. If you knew that your child had this gene (and this can be determined with a blood test), you could give your child a low-salt diet and perhaps spare him or her from developing high blood pressure as an adult.

Cells that eat better communicate better. Cells communicate by producing substances that affect other cells. For example, cells produce hormones, which carry messages to other cells and organs and tell them what to do. Hormones are involved in many, many functions in the body. For example, certain hormones help the body deal with stress. Others regulate appetite, affect sexual development, and even stimulate emotions.

We know that hormones are greatly influenced by nutrition. This is most obvious in the realm of insulin sensitivity. Insulin is the hormone that tells cells to let in glucose, which they need for energy. Studies of infant animals show that too much sugar can result in cells' becoming resistant to insulin in adulthood and can lead to Type 2 diabetes.

Cells also communicate with each other using neurotransmitters. Neurotransmitters are chemicals that nerve cells use to talk with each other, especially in the brain and the intestinal tract. The healthier the nutrients in the blood, the better the quality of the neurotransmitters. Since neurotransmitters affect thinking and emotions, they are an important route by which nutrition influences your child's quality of life.

Cells that are fed better are built better. Cells are surrounded by a membrane that is like a skin. The cell receives messages through the membrane, thanks to millions of receptor sites for hormones

FEEDING YOUR FAMILY'S GENETIC QUIRKS

Different families have different quirky genes, meaning genes that increase the chances of getting a certain illness such as a particular type of cancer or diabetes. How nutrition might affect an individual's genes is called nutrigenetics. We believe that someday part of a general health checkup will be blood tests to identify these genetic quirks so that the doctor can make a more compelling case for prescribing a diet and lifestyle specifically tailored to each individual. We believe in the not-so-distant future, we will be having this conversation with a family: "From the blood tests it seems that your child has a tendency to develop Type 2 diabetes. Here is a list of changes I want you to make in how your family eats and lives. They should greatly lower your child's chance of ever developing diabetes."

The good news is that having a particular gene associated with cardiovascular illness, diabetes, or cancer does not mean you will automatically get the illness associated with it. In order for these genetic quirks to translate into an illness, they have to be ex-

and neurotransmitters. These receptor sites are like microscopic locks, and the chemical messengers that circulate throughout the body are like the keys. Certain keys fit certain locks, and when the key fits into the lock, something good happens. If the receptor sites are defective, which can happen when a child is not getting the right nutrients, the cell is not able to receive and act on certain messages.

The cell membrane has another job as well. It is to be selective about what it lets into the cell and what it keeps out. When the cell membrane is constructed properly with the right nutrient-building blocks, it lets in the good stuff from the bloodstream and keeps out the bad stuff such as pollutants and toxins.

The cell membranes are composed mainly of fats, especially

pressed, meaning a number of factors have to combine to cause problems. Whether or not a genetic quirk is expressed or repressed can be influenced greatly by lifestyle and nutrition.

At present, we may not know all of our children's genetic quirks or when or even whether these genetic tendencies will result in a full-blown illness. The nutritional program in this book covers all the bases. Having thoroughly reviewed credible science linking early feeding practices with risk reduction of later illnesses, we can say that the nutritional changes we ask you to make in your family will lower the chances that your children will get any of the major diseases.

One day I (Bill) was explaining the concept of nutrigenetics and quirky genes to twelve-year-old Ashley, a patient in our medical practice. After hearing about this interesting subject, she decided to do a science project about it and asked me, "Dr. Bill, does that mean that food can fool the genes? We have a lot of people with high blood pressure in our family. Could what I eat turn on or turn off my genes for high blood pressure?" Ashley got it!

the good fats, such as the omega 3's in seafood. Bad fats, like hydrogenated oils, act like molecular misfits and clog the receptor sites on the cell membrane. The type of fat in a child's diet affects how well cells are able to communicate with one another and protect themselves from toxins. This is one of the reasons that throughout this book we emphasize how important it is to feed your child a right-fat diet. Getting the right fats is critical to having healthy brain cells and healthy cells in the rest of the body. (For more about fats and brain health, see chapter 4, Feed Your Family a Right-Fat Diet.)

Cells that are fed right produce energy more efficiently. Within each cell are tiny boxes called mitochondria, which create and store energy needed for the cell to work and reproduce. These little energy generators are sensitive to nutrition. Feed the cell a junk-food diet and cells can't make energy very efficiently. This is one of the reasons why fatigue frequently accompanies poor nutrition. One of the first changes children on our nutritional program report is "I have so much more energy."

Dr. Jim learned firsthand the connection between food and energy:

> *In my four years at college I ate in the cafeteria, mostly mass-produced, processed foods. I spent every evening after dinner feeling a bit foggy and tired. I never realized that these feelings were not normal until I graduated, began eating better food, and started feeling better!*

The concepts of metabolic programming and nutrigenetics seem to play a part in the childhood obesity epidemic. Obesity researchers believe humans have adapted so-called thrifty genes, genes that turn on when food is plentiful so that the body can store extra food as needed calories in case famine occurs, thus enabling a more efficient use of food resources. These thrifty genes were probably a survival mechanism in the early days of humanity, when feast and famine were realities of life. The fear of famine no longer exists in developed countries, yet the thrifty genes remain. When you overfeed a child, you turn on those thrifty genes, increasing the chances that the child will become a calorie storer and, consequently, have a lifelong tendency to be overfat and to have more difficulty shedding those extra fat rolls. On the other

---

GROWING HEALTHY HEARTS

One of the biggest breakthroughs in what we know about metabolic programming is that early eating practices can set a child up for a long life of healthy heart function or a shorter and sicker life overshadowed by cardiovascular disease. The body reacts to a diet full of junk carbs and junk fats by producing excess amounts of harmful substances, especially inflammatory substances called cytokines, which damage the lining of the blood vessels. This lining is called the endothelium, and it operates like a built-in pharmacy for the cardiovascular system. It secretes substances that repair the damage done by inflammation, relax the arteries, and keep fat from building up in the blood vessels. But if you don't feed the endothelium properly, it can't do its job. In early childhood, a difference between the "pure kids," whose arteries are smooth inside like Teflon, and the junk-food-eating children, whose arteries are like Velcro on the inside, is not detectable. Both have good enough blood flow — for now. But eventually the clogged, stiff arteries of the poorly nourished children will make them more prone to high blood pressure, strokes, and heart attacks as adults. Which kind of arteries do you want your child to grow?

hand, raising a lean child, as you will learn about in chapter 9, keeps those thrifty genes from being expressed.

Don't raise an iBod. The concept of metabolic programming is particularly relevant to the development of a child's immune system. Scientists are finding that many illnesses (e.g., diabetes, cardiovascular disease, dementia, asthma) are the result of an immune system that has gone awry and is attacking cells in the body as if they were foreign invaders. These cells become inflamed and damaged. This inflammation is at the heart of "-itis" diseases, such as colitis and arthritis. It also plays a role in the development of high blood sugar, high cholesterol, and high blood pressure. In fact, we have coined a term for children who grow up with this problem — "iBods" (see page 206). Having the right nutrients in the body helps prevent the immune system from going haywire. The right nutrients also help cells repair themselves when something goes wrong.

HOW THIS METABOLIC MESS HAPPENED

You may wonder how there came to be such a metabolic mismatch between what we eat and what our bodies can process. Here, in a nutshell, is how it happened. Over the course of millions of years, the human body has adapted to eat the food that has been most available: meat from wild animals, seafood, and a variety of plant foods — grains, fruits, and vegetables. The body developed an efficient storage system to store energy as fat when food was plentiful and to use this stored fat when food was scarce. Note that the natural diet for humans did not contain hydrogenated fats, fiberless grains, high-fructose corn syrup, or artificial flavorings, colorings, and preservatives. Meat was lean, relatively free of saturated, harmful fats, and rich in healthful omega-3 fats. Then came "progress." Game that was previously wild started being farmed in pens, and the cows, pigs, and chickens consumed less healthy food all day, as did the penned-up fish. As a result, the meat and seafood became higher in bad fats and lower in good fats. Consequently, the penned-up animals, with their junk-food diets, became more prone to infectious diseases, so they were injected with antibiotics, hormones, and whatever chemicals were necessary to keep them alive and fat.

Then along came more agricultural "progress," in the form of food processing. Nutrients that the body needs were removed for the sake of a longer shelf life and appearance, and artificial ingredients were added to "replace" the lost nutrients. As a result, the good fats in domesticated meat have become unhealthful, as have the sugars in processed grains. Nutrition researchers call this factory-processed nutrition "genetically unknown food," meaning our genes don't recognize this stuff as real food.

On the outside we may seem to have adapted to this changing food supply. In developed countries, food is plentiful, and kids grow. But the human species has not had time to adapt its genetic, digestive, and metabolic mechanisms to handle factory-made food, and on the inside, our bodies have paid a price. Our hormones are just a little bit off, our body chemistry is out of balance, and there is a gradual increase in wear and tear (i.e., inflammation), which we call "factory fallout" from fake food. Over the years, this has taken its toll on children's bodies, and they have started being programmed toward diseases such as Type 2 diabetes, cardiovascular disease, and all the "-itis" illnesses. Kids and adults need diets more like those of our ancestors. These are the foods that our bodies were designed to use.

A wise schoolteacher in one of our children's classes said to her students: "If it's packaged food and your mother didn't package it, it's probably junk." This bit of teacher wisdom summarizes the whole problem with children's nutrition. Children's bodies were never designed to metabolize processed food, and they pay a price for doing so. How do we get our children's bodies back on the right nutritional track?

SHAPE YOUNG TASTES AND CHANGE YOUNG CRAVINGS

Shaping young tastes and changing young cravings are important concepts in reclaiming our children's nutritional health. Over the past ten years, research in many university nutrition centers has confirmed what food-savvy parents have long suspected: The healthier children eat in the early years, the healthier they are likely to eat — and be — as adults.

Children believe what their parents tell them. They copy what their parents do, and they carry into adulthood their knowledge about the way their parents did things. Some of this life wisdom may be reevaluated by the time kids become adults, and some parental beliefs may ultimately be rejected. But much of what kids learn in the early years of life will influence their behavior for as long as they live.

This is one reason why it is so important for parents to feed their children healthy meals. Children's beliefs about what to eat are formed early, and the ideas about food that are learned in childhood influence our eating patterns and health as adults. The memories of our early meals, and the feelings of security and comfort that come with being part of a family, become part of our associations with food. When children are fed nutritious foods, later in life they seek out those same healthy foods as adults to help them feel happy and secure.

One of the most important features of metabolic programming is that it helps maintain good eating habits. Cells that are programmed by good nutrition to function in a good way "remember" what is good for them. They work with other cells, releasing hormones and using and storing energy in ways that prompt the body to crave more of the nutrients that will keep it on the right track. It's as if the cells memorize the recipe for health that they learn in the early years and continue to send signals to the brain that say, "This food is good for me. Feed me more." The cells are accustomed to a high standard of living, and they support and reward the body when it maintains high nutritional standards. Bottom line: Child doesn't like broccoli, child eats broccoli a while, child likes broccoli.

SHAPE YOUNG ATTITUDES

Of course, kids and grown-ups may not always listen to the "eat good food" messages that their bodies are sending them. Other messages sometimes get in the way: "Junk food is fun." "Cake is how we celebrate." "Cookies make me happy." Attitude is an important part of developing good eating habits. You want your child to grow up believing that we feel good when we are healthy, and good health comes from making wise food choices. A "pure mom" of a "pure kid" told us this story about her five-year-old daughter:

> *One night my mother was babysitting Lauren. While they were changing pajamas together, Lauren noticed some rolls of fat around Grandma's waist. Lauren asked, "How did you get those?" Grandma replied, "I made some poor food choices." The following week Lauren and I saw her other grandma, who had put on a lot of weight since the last time Lauren had seen her. Lauren whispered to me, "Grandma made poor food choices!"*

At five years of age Lauren had already learned a valuable lesson in life: Poor food choices leave a lasting impression on the body.

IT'S NEVER TOO LATE TO START!

While there is a unique window of opportunity for shaping your children's food preferences during the early years, it's not an all-or-nothing situation. Metabolic programming can be very effective at shaping tastes at any age. Your body is constantly making new cells, no matter how old you are. It's never too late to teach those cells what's good for them.

Children — and adults — often have a hard time distinguishing between healthy messages from the body about eating and less healthy messages. For example, eating sweets triggers the release of the "happy hormone," serotonin. Someone who eats a lot of sweets might crave a cookie or a candy bar in a stressful situation, because his body believes that the high-carb treat will make him feel better. Unfortunately, the feel-good effect of dipping into the chocolate chip cookies won't last long. The person's blood sugar will zoom up and then quickly drop, leaving him restless, anxious, and craving more high-carb foods.

It's up to the brain to recognize and control cravings that are not good for the body. Children's brains learn how to control cravings by listening to both messages from the body and messages from the outside, from parents and other trusted authority figures. Positive metabolic programming gets the cells used to an optimal level of nutrients for optimal health, so they continue to send out neurochemicals that guide the child's cravings toward continued healthy eating. The example of healthy eating provided by parents, along with the messages that parents share with their children about good foods, help kids tune in to their bodies and tune out unhealthy messages that they get from the media and their peers.

The gut feeling: good or bad? Guess where most of the feel-good neurochemicals in your body reside. Surprisingly, it's not the brain but the gut. Most of the body's serotonin is produced in the nerves of the intestinal lining. (There is some neurochemical truth behind the idea of "gut feelings.") So it's no surprise that eating well can make you feel good — emotionally as well as physically. All those nerve endings are busy transmitting information, which is why scientists use the term "gut brain." When a real food enters the gut, nerves in the digestive system sense, "Ah! The right stuff!"

Sadly, kids can grow up craving the wrong kind of food. If a child grows up metabolically programmed toward junk food, the cells get used to this level of nutrients and regard this way of eating as the norm. The body ends up craving the foods that contribute to its own poor health. This craving quirk is especially true for what is called our sweet tooth. Instead of craving the natural sweetness of fruit (e.g., blueberries added to plain yogurt), the junk-food addict craves the artificially sweetened, bright pink yogurt made in the food factory. "Pure kids" tell me that sugar-sweetened, artificially flavored beverages make them feel yucky. Yet junk-food-eaters often say, "It doesn't bother me!" That's the problem. The effects of eating junk food should bother a child, and if they don't, that child's tastes and cravings need to be re-shaped in a healthier direction.

Parents in our practice call the relationship between what their children eat and how they feel "the connection." During their children's preschool years, we talk to them a lot about shaping their kids' tastes to prefer the good feeling they get from eating healthy food. Even when their children are as young as five, parents often report, "You know, Dr. Sears, she's finally making the connection between what she eats and how she feels."

A TALE OF TWO EATERS ON
TWO DIFFERENT NUTRITIONAL TRACKS

Meet two real kids from our practice: a "pure kid" (PK) and a "junk-food kid" (JFK). PK's "pure mom" (PM) belonged to a group we call in our practice "high investors." They realize that raising kids who turn out well is just like any investment. You plan a wise course of action and you invest early if you want a good return in the future. Later on, you sit back and enjoy seeing how your investment has paid off. PM considered giving her child the gift of health one of the best long-term investments she could make.

In the early years she figured out an important nutritional investment strategy: Determine which foods you want your child to acquire a taste for, and feed her those. She started out by breastfeeding PK. Then, beginning at six months, she made PK's baby food from scratch. By one year of age, PK was eating small bits of wild salmon, tofu, avocado, hummus, flaxseed meal, and puréed fresh fruits and vegetables. In fact, by one year of age, PK was eating almost the same fare PM served the rest of the family. PK grew up liking the feeling of being not too full but never really hungry, so she became a *grazer* — nibbling on nutritious foods throughout the day besides enjoying the scheduled meals with the family. And, realizing that all children have a sweet tooth (after all, breast milk is naturally sweet), PM served PK yogurt sweetened with mashed blueberries. When PK was invited to parties, PM took along her favorite berries for cake time.

By three years of age, PK noticed she was eating foods that were different from what her friends ate. When other kids were snacking on chips at the park, PM simply said, "We don't eat that in our family," as she opened a bag of whole-grain pita chips. By age five PK started to notice fast-food restaurants, so PM would repeat, "We don't eat at those places in our family." When pressed, she would add, "Because I love you, I won't let you put that stuff in your body. Instead, we'll go to the farmer's market for a treat."

When PK went to school, she was exposed to more junk food, including treats at birthday parties and school cafeteria lunches. Being a kid, naturally she had to try some of this stuff. When she did, she noticed how it made her feel. Because her taste buds and the lining of her gut had been programmed to enjoy the taste and texture of natural foods, the chemically processed foods left a bad taste in her mouth and a bad feeling in her gut. PK had learned that eating is supposed to be pleasurable. Her early programming set her up to learn this important lesson: Eat good food, feel good. Eat bad food, feel bad.

PM was careful not to make bad food forbidden food. (Kids seem attracted to anything "forbidden.") She took the positive approach and simply presented healthy food with the attitude that this was what smart people eat. Junk food was just that — junk. Sometimes she'd add, "Your body is beautiful, and it deserves good grow foods." PK liked the term "grow food" because it made her sound big and strong. When her friends were sick and missed school or playdates, PM was quick to point out, "Grow foods fight germs, so you don't get sick as often."

NUTSHELL

Good food makes you feel good; junk food makes you feel junky.

PK enjoyed shopping with her mother, who treated the supermarket like a giant nutritional classroom. PM taught PK, "We shop mainly the perimeter. That's where the grow foods are."

When passing the junk-food aisle, PM added, "And that's an aisle we just don't go down. It has foods that keep you from growing."

When PK asked for food that featured her favorite cartoon characters on the package, her mother quickly intervened, "Sorry, honey, that's not real food." By the time she was nine, PK realized that manufacturers try to trick kids into eating foods that are not good for them by using advertising to make these foods seem cool. By the age of ten, PK was playing the I Spy game (on her own) by looking for the "good words" like "whole grains" on the cereal box label and finding the small print with the "bad words" like "high-fructose corn syrup" and "hydrogenated," and all the color-number symbols, such as red #40.

NUTSHELL
Grow foods keep you well;
junk food can make you sick.

PM realized that variety is the spice — and the health — of life. So every now and then, the family would eat out at an ethnic restaurant. PM never let her kids order from kids' menus full of hot dogs and chicken nuggets. When PK asked her mom why, PM replied, "Because that's junk food. You deserve better. You can order real food off the adult menu." That made her feel big and important. So everyone in the family ordered a different dish, with varying degrees of spiciness, encouraging PK to try "just two bites" of even the weirdest-looking or -tasting foods. Because whole foods are naturally filling, PK seldom overate. She felt just right, neither too full nor hungry. As a result, she stayed lean and grew healthier.

Let's contrast PK with JFK — junk-food kid — who had spent the early years of his life eating mostly food out of a jar, a box, or a fast-food outlet. Sadly, he believed that this was what food was supposed to taste like. He didn't always feel comfortable after eating, but he assumed that this was how people feel after they eat. Because he ate a lot of processed foods, from which the fiber and other grow-food nutrients had been removed, he

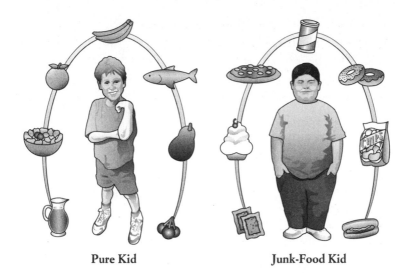

Pure Kid　　　　　　　**Junk-Food Kid**

never felt satisfied, so he tended to overeat. Because the natural "I'm full" signals that the stomach sends to the brain never functioned properly for JFK, he never learned to eat appropriate amounts of food. Because the processed sugar in his diet went into and out of his bloodstream quickly, he constantly craved sweets. Gradually, the overeating of junk food made him overfat. JFK grew — parts of him overgrew — especially around the middle.

On the outside, PK and JFK both seemed to be growing, but inside, at the cellular, molecular, genetic, and biochemical levels, they were very different. JFK's bloodstream was filled with harmful biochemical substances that his body was producing in reaction to his junk-food diet. His system was full of inflammatory chemicals, increasing the wear and tear on all his tissues. His bloodstream was full of junk fats, which little by little were deposited on his increasingly narrowing blood vessels. Not so for PK's bloodstream. Unlike the lining of JFK's blood vessels, which was rough like Velcro, the lining of her blood vessels was smooth like Teflon. Her blood sugar levels were more stable, as were her moods; JFK's blood sugar was up and down all the time, and so were his moods. JFK's joints became more susceptible to wear and tear from all the extra stuff in his bloodstream that shouldn't have been there and all the waste products that were produced when his immune system tried to fight them. As he got older, each organ aged too fast from wear and tear and insufficient blood flow.

Which of these two tracks is your child on? Which child do you have at your dinner table? Now is the time to make your kids "pure kids."

TEN WAYS TO SHAPE YOUNG TASTES

Tastes and cravings are learned in the body and in the brain but influenced mostly by cultural eating practices. While American children learn to love hamburgers, children in China or India learn to love other foods. Here are time-tested ways to shape your children's tastes from birth onward.

1. Breastfeed As Often and for As Long As Possible

Almost everyone now knows that human milk is the gold standard for infant nutrition. In fact, the positive effects of breastfeeding on adult health is the prime example of how early metabolic programming can protect against adult diseases such as diabetes and high blood pressure. You can lower the incidence of just about every disease by breastfeeding. And the effect is dose related: the longer and more exclusively you breastfeed your children, the greater the health benefits. New research has traced some of these health-promoting effects to the fact that breastfed children grow up with lower and more stable insulin levels. Growing up with too high and unstable insulin levels in the bloodstream produces an unfavorable biological environment, so the body and brain cannot grow optimally. Other benefits of breast milk include its heart-healthy fats and immune boosters and the gut-friendly quality of human milk protein. Here are some specific ways that breastfeeding can shape young tastes.

It promotes a good gut feeling. Breast milk is known as an "easy-in, easy-out" food. Its perfect balance of the right kinds of fats, proteins, and carbohydrates makes it easy on the intestines. Breastfed babies begin life associating good gut feelings with eating. They also associate the warmth and comfort of being close to Mom with mealtime. Could there be a better food-mood connection?

It provides ideal metabolic programming. Breast milk gives babies the best possible metabolic programming in the first weeks and months of life. The unique brain-building fats in breast milk help infant brains grow to be the best they can be. The many immunological factors in human milk help the baby's own immune system to develop. It's interesting to note that breastfeeding during infancy is associated with a lower lifelong risk of many diseases thought to be caused by immune system dysfunction, including juvenile diabetes, multiple sclerosis, and Crohn's disease.

It introduces foods of the culture. Breast milk plays an important part in transmitting taste preferences for different cultures' cuisines. A mother's milk actually carries flavors from the foods she eats. Breastfeeding gets babies ready to enjoy the more flavorful foods their families eat. Variations in the taste of the milk from day to day prepare baby for a varied diet in the years ahead.

It prevents overeating. Breastfed babies seem to grow up being better able to decide how much to eat. Studies have shown that children who are breastfed are less likely to be obese in adolescence. Because breast milk is emptied faster from the stomach, breastfed babies naturally tend to eat more frequently, but smaller amounts. As a result, they get accustomed to the wise nutritional principle of grazing. (You will learn a lot about the health benefits of grazing in chapter 6.) When feeding at the breast, babies decide for themselves when they are hungry and when they are satisfied. You can get a formula-fed baby to finish that last half-ounce in the bottle, even if his tummy is full. A breastfed baby simply stops sucking when she has had enough.

One of the most exciting new areas of research on early metabolic programming is about how breastfed and formula-fed infants become biochemically different. For example, breastfed infants have higher leptin levels in their bloodstream. Leptin is a potent appetite-regulating hormone. Researchers have long theorized that because breast milk is a medium-cholesterol diet, whereas infant formula contains little cholesterol, breastfed infants learn to metabolize dietary cholesterol better early in life, and thus grow up to have fewer problems with cardiovascular disease. Although it's hard to design a study to prove this theory, scientists are constantly discovering new and interesting ways in which breastfeeding really does make a difference to children's health. (For more about the long-term benefits of breastfeeding, see our book *The Breastfeeding Book,* Little, Brown, 2000.)

2. Serve Fresh or Frozen Baby and Toddler Food

Introduce your baby to the flavor of fresh foods right from the start. The less canned formula and jarred food your baby and toddler eats, the better. When toddlers eat fresh food, they learn what real food tastes like in the mouth and feels like in the gut.

They learn to enjoy a greater variety of flavors and textures. These early encounters with solid food are a window of opportunity for shaping young tastes. If your baby and toddler eats only freshly prepared, unsalted, and unsweetened foods, your child will prefer these foods and be more likely to reject salty, sugar-sweetened junk foods. It's as simple as that.

Infants and children do have a built-in preference for sweet-tasting foods. Breast milk is naturally sweet, and studies of newborns have demonstrated that babies just a few days old prefer sugar water to plain water. Babies' inborn preference for sweet food is nature's way of ensuring that they like to drink the good stuff — their mother's milk — that helps them grow. Human milk and the healthy fresh foods that older babies enjoy such as bananas and other ripe fruits have a natural sweetness in them that is not overwhelming or artificial. A baby whose favorite foods are Mother's milk and squishy bananas probably won't go on to enjoy beverages sweetened with massive amounts of sugar, corn syrup, or artificial sweeteners. These foods will taste sickeningly sweet when compared with the naturally sweetened foods he learned to love early in life. When artificial sweets hit the programmed receptors in the lining of his gut, they trigger an internal biochemical alarm that registers as "yucky." On the other hand, children who grow up with a steady diet of sweetened, salted, and greasy fast foods don't register these foods as "yucky," because they have become used to them.

One of the most brilliant but nutritionally destructive baby snack foods we've ever seen are the dried puffed vegetable snacks. They come in a convenient can and have the word "veggies" right on the front. What better snack could there possibly be for a child? You can take them anywhere! Sure, there may be veggies in the ingredients, but think about this: You are teaching your baby that veggies (and all snack foods, for that matter) shouldn't taste fresh and juicy and real. Your baby is learning that food should taste like chips. If *babies* grow up snacking on artificial crackers and puffs all day, it's no wonder they don't want to eat real fruits and veggies as they get older.

3. Graze on Grow Foods

One of the most common problems parents of one- to three-year-olds raise during routine checkups is that their child doesn't eat enough. We believe one of the main reasons parents think their child doesn't eat enough is that they expect their child to eat three good-sized meals each day. But young children have tiny tummies, about the size of their fists. They feel more comfortable grazing on mini-meals throughout the day. Grazing is actually healthier for them.

Not only do most kids eat too much junk food, most older kids eat too much — period! This is true of adults as well. "Supersize me," we say at restaurants. We have come to view large portions as the norm, and this has turned us into a nation of habitual overeaters. There are sensors in the stomach called stretch receptors. When the stomach is filled with a certain volume of food, these receptors signal the brain, "Stop, you've eaten enough!" Research on animals suggests that those who eat too much end up with stretched stomachs that wait longer to send the stop signal. A grazer, someone who eats small portions more frequently, gets used to feeling satisfied with less. By offering your child fre-

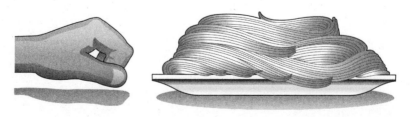

A portion that is bigger than your child's fist is too much!

quent mini-meals throughout the day, you can literally shape the size and portion expectations of your child's tummy. (See also chapter 6, Raise a Grazer.)

4. Avoid the "Terrible Threes"

Don't feed your child foods containing these three artificial additives:

- high-fructose corn syrup
- hydrogenated oils, or "trans fats"
- any color additive with a number symbol attached to it (e.g., blue #1, yellow #5, red #40)

These are three easy-to-remember ways to recognize foods that merit the label "junk food." Not only are these ingredients themselves unhealthy for your child, but any packaged food that contains them is likely to be something you don't want your kids to eat. If you make this one change — avoiding foods that contain any of these three ingredients — you will have gone 90 percent of the way toward de-junking your child's diet. Food packagers actually add ingredients that are designed to entice children to crave a particular "mouth feel." Remember the chip advertising slogan "Bet you can't eat just one!"

5. Serve Nutrient-Dense Foods

Your baby or young child's first foods should be grow foods, which we also like to call "superfoods." These are the foods you most want your children to eat when they are older, so it's important that they learn to like them and see them as a part of their everyday diet. On page 34 you learned how the nutrients in foods may interact with a child's genetic makeup, especially if the child has a genetic quirk predisposing him to a certain disease. Since we can't know all the genetic quirks our children may have, it's wise to cover all the bases.

Grow foods are fresh foods or packaged foods that have undergone minimal amounts of processing. They are foods you eat as close to their natural state as possible. They do not contain artificial or factory-added ingredients, and they are nutrient dense — they pack a lot of nutrition into a relatively small volume of food. Nutrient-dense foods are different from calorie-dense foods, those that pack a lot of calories into a small volume of food. Studies have shown that children who are habitually fed nutrient-dense foods tend to prefer them and are less likely to overeat than children who are fed a steady diet of nutrient-poor foods.

Young children who are served nutrient-dense foods from an early age do learn to prefer these foods. We have seen this with our newest grandchild, Ashton, the ultimate "pure kid" of a "pure mom." One night as we were preparing to babysit fourteen-month-old Ashton, our daughter Hayden laid out her daughter's snacks and dinner: wild salmon, bell pepper, cooked spinach, tofu, avocado, and hummus. Ashton is now three, and the other day when we visited Hayden, we watched her put some leaves of Swiss chard into Ashton's fruit-and-yogurt smoothie. Ashton craves (or at least accepts) foods that are shunned by typical toddlers because her tastes have already been shaped toward these grow foods. And she's already beginning to make the connection "I eat right, I feel right."

NUTSHELL

When your children are especially hungry, be sure to serve them grow foods rather than junk foods. Children tend to develop preferences for foods that they eat when they are most hungry, since these foods are perceived as the most satisfying.

THE TOP 12 SUPERFOODS OR GROW FOODS

Help your child grow a taste for these nutrient-dense foods: *

- avocados
- beans, kidney
- blueberries
- eggs
- flaxseed meal
- ground nuts, nut butters (to prevent choking, spread nut butter in a thin layer; avoid giving whole nuts to children under the age of three)
- oatmeal
- salmon, wild
- spinach
- tofu
- tomatoes
- yogurt, organic

Honorable Mention

- broccoli
- lentils
- olive oil
- oranges
- papaya
- pink grapefruit
- poultry, organic
- sweet potatoes

* According to our calculations, these foods contain more health-enriching nutrients than are found in equal volumes or equal numbers of calories of other foods. Almost all fruits and vegetables could be included in this list of superfoods. (See chapter 5 for more about grow foods.)

Because Ashton is too young to safely eat nuts and seeds, I grind foods like almonds, sunflower seeds, and flaxseeds in a coffee grinder and sprinkle them on her cereal or yogurt. This gets her used to their taste.

6. Model Healthy Eating Habits

Studies have shown that children tend to develop food preferences and eating habits similar to their mothers' preferences and habits. (Sorry, dads, that's just the way it is — and maybe it's just as well!) If you present nutritious foods as the norm ("This is what we eat") and eat them yourself, your children will eat them, too. It's as simple as that. As much as possible, keep your preschool and school-age children from exposure to junk food and advertisements for junk food. There is an interesting study of four hundred British children aged four to eleven who were shown videos of superheroes enjoying fruits and vegetables. These children consumed greater amounts of fruits and vegetables than usual after watching these videos.

7. Shape, Don't Control!

Studies have shown that rigidly restricting children's access to certain foods focuses more attention on these foods and increases children's desire to eat them. Parents who try to *control* their children's eating habits end up with kids who are more likely to overeat and to eat the wrong kinds of foods. Also, children who are raised in families with highly controlling and restrictive attitudes toward eating tend to have a higher level of dissatisfaction with their bodies. Clearly, trying to control your older child's eating habits could trigger an eating disorder.

Instead, think in terms of *shaping* your child's food preferences. "Shaping" means providing your child with opportunities to make wise choices, and directing and redirecting behavior in ways that help your child learn to be in charge of himself. It's good discipline, applied to food. Shaping is like gardening. You plant the seed, and while you can't control how fast the plant grows or when it blooms, you can pull the weeds around it and water it and prune it to help it grow more beautifully. Don't coerce your children into eating or penalize them for not eating. Don't make threats such as "You must eat your vegetables or you can't watch TV." Long-term studies have shown that this is a for-sure way to keep your child from liking vegetables. It's okay, though, to set some priorities: "Grow foods before fun foods!" Just make sure there's a tried-and-true favorite grow food on the table so that your child is guaranteed to enjoy eating at least one grow food on the way to a healthy dessert.

8. Surround Your Child with Nutritious Foods

What's in your pantry? Studies show that preschool-age children are more likely to eat the foods that are most accessible. When children see a bowl of fruit or a platter of raw vegetables sitting on the table as snack food, this is what they will eat. They won't go looking in the pantry for junk food. (This strategy works on moms and dads, too.) Restock your pantry with the foods you want them to like. These will become their familiar foods, or "family foods," the ones that are the norm for your family.

One reason fast-food restaurants and junk-food snacks are so popular is that they are very accessible — no chopping, no cooking, no dishes to wash. Just place your order at the drive-through window, or pop open the plastic wrapper. Reminders that these foods are available can be found almost everywhere. Tastes are shaped not only in mouths and guts but also in little eyes. Make sure your kids see healthy food when they walk into your kitchen.

9. Expose Your Child to a Variety of *New* Foods

We often hear parents complain, "My child just won't try new foods." Food researchers believe that an aversion to trying new foods is a built-in safety mechanism. Back when food was hunted or gathered from the fields and forests, it was smart to be cautious about trying new foods. Some could be poisonous — most likely the ones that were not sweet and that had a funny taste. Familiar foods, the ones the family ate all the time, were the safest. Experts in infant feeding and development believe that this innate fear is what causes a toddler to go through a stage of finicky or picky eating.

Whatever the reasons behind food aversions, getting children out of a food-choice rut can be frustrating. But it's important to try. Your children need to eat a variety of foods to get the right balance of vitamins, minerals, carbohydrates, fats, and proteins. It takes creative marketing to get children to experiment with new tastes and textures. Here are some new-food marketing tips:

Start early. Studies show that new foods are most likely to be accepted between two and three years of age. This is why it's important to introduce a variety of grow foods during that window of opportunity in the early years.

He's more likely to try a new food if I sit him on my lap and put the new food on my plate.

Go small. Begin with small amounts, such as 1 or 2 teaspoons. That way if your child doesn't like the new food, no one gets frustrated and you don't worry about wasting good food.

Make hunger work for you. Children are most likely to accept new foods when they are especially hungry. Try offering new foods at times when your child is most hungry, such as at a midafternoon snack. A new food can be a fun novelty at snacktime. At mealtime, when other choices are available, a child may be less likely to try something new.

Hide the food. Be sneaky. Hide a new food in a tried-and-true favorite food. Use a larger amount of the favorite food (e.g., four parts familiar food to one part new food), and each time you serve this combination, gradually increase the proportion of the new food. One of our children loved blueberries, so we put a pile of blueberries over a little plain yogurt. She gradually began to mix the blueberries into the yogurt. For one of our other children, we camouflaged avocado with peanut butter. Using the favorite food as camouflage over the new food will often introduce children to the taste of a new food in a less intimidating way, since it's partnered with their favorite. Children often prefer a combo to individual foods.

Repeat, repeat, repeat! Try the "rule of ten." Studies from the Department of Nutrition at Penn State University have shown that repeated exposure (usually between ten and twenty times) to a new food eventually leads most children to accept it. So if your five-year-old shuns broccoli, don't give up after only three or four tries. Keep offering it in different presentations (e.g., steamed or raw with dip, drizzled with olive oil, covered with cheese, mixed with pasta, in soup and salads). Eventually your child will eat broccoli because it's there, letting him know "this is what we eat."

Play copycat. When you eat something that you are trying to get your child to like, let your child see you eat it with gusto. Children like to copy their parents, and they're curious when it seems they might be missing out on something fun. If there's something you want your child to try, eat it right in front of him without actually offering it to him. He may try the new food simply because you are eating it. Of course, you may have to fake it if you want your child to learn to like something you don't enjoy. Parents who want to shape their children's tastes toward healthy food often find themselves eating better when their kids are around. If a parent says, "No way am I eating that," the child won't eat it either.

When she sees me eat it, she wants to try it, too.

Try the two-bite deal. In our family we encourage our children, "Take two bites. If you like it, fine. If you don't, you don't have to eat it. You can try it again another time." If it's really a no, don't push it.

Be enthusiastic. Introduce the new food with enthusiasm and excitement. Make an appreciative face and say, "Yum, good!" Play show and tell: Name it, show it, describe it, take a bite yourself, and talk about how tasty it is. If you child rejects the food, don't force the issue. Research shows that children are more likely to accept new foods when they are simply exposed to them rather than forced to eat them. Continue to serve the food, and one day your child may surprise you by asking for it. Be sure to present new foods positively. One time we were filling our plates from a buffet of unusual ethnic foods. A mother in front of us said to her curious five-year-old, "You can try it, but you probably won't like it." That comment put a damper on her child's enthusiasm for new foods. Children are more likely to try new foods willingly when the atmosphere around the table is happy and positive.

Be aware of a food-refusal quirk called conditioned aversion, in which a child associates eating a certain food with a bad gut feeling. I (Dr. Bill) still remember the time as a young child when I ate a hamburger, and the ketchup on it tasted awful. Later that day I developed food poisoning and felt awful. I don't know whether it was the hamburger or the ketchup, but I wouldn't touch either one for a couple years. Preschool children are particularly vulnerable to gastrointestinal illnesses and memories of bad food, and parents need to be especially vigilant about food safety at this stage. A strong aversion to a particular food may also be a sign of allergy or food intolerance.

Try tricks. You may be able to trick young children into eating a food they don't like. Dr. Bob found an easy way to get his child to love carrots:

> *We were at a dinner and magic show, and our three-year-old was finished with his very small dinner. When he wasn't looking, I put a carrot from my plate on his. He noticed it, and curious, he looked at me. "It's a magic carrot," I said. "The magician made it magically appear on your plate!" He ate it up, along with another ten carrots that "magically" appeared when he wasn't looking. Now he eats his "magic carrots" anytime we serve them at home.*

Co-cook. Children are more likely to eat foods that they have helped to prepare. If they've invested a lot of time and energy in helping to make the meal, they are going to want to sample their handiwork. They may even try the new food during the preparation and enjoy it.

Try peer pressure. Invite other children to your home for a meal — kids who you know eat a variety of foods that you want your child to learn to enjoy. When children see other kids, especially their friends or slightly older kids whom they look up to, eating a new food, they are more likely to try it.

Go ethnic! Visit ethnic restaurants when your children are young to introduce them to a wide variety of foods. Try Indian, Asian, and Middle Eastern restaurants. Be careful, though: American Chinese food is often full of fat, sugar, and MSG. Children are attracted to novelty. Like the experience of looking at all the toys in the toy store, being exposed to a variety of unfamiliar foods

> **NUTSHELL**
> **Shapes Make Shaping Tastes Easier.**
> Kids are fascinated by fun shapes. Cutting foods into various shapes, such as stars and circles, gets kids to focus on the shape rather than the unfamiliarity of the new food.

piques their interest. Of course, be sure to show that you enjoy these outings yourself, since children's acceptance of new and unusual foods often depends upon watching the reaction of others. It's healthy for children to grow up with a cuisine curiosity. Hummus is a great shaping food because it contains spices, olive oil, and garbanzo beans — all foods you want your kids to like.

Shaping children's tastes and food preferences is a lot like teaching them a second language at a young age: exposure, exposure, exposure is everything. What "food language" do you want your children to learn?

10. Enjoy Happy Meals

Eating is supposed to be pleasurable. The more friendly the atmosphere around the table, the more likely your children are to try new foods prepared in different ways, and also to eat appropriate amounts — not too little and not too much.

"My kids just won't eat healthy food," you may complain. What good is all this nutritional advice if your kids won't eat what you serve? For those of you with infants less than one year of age, following our advice will be a "piece of cake." Just get them on the right track from the start (which also means getting yourselves on this same train), and they'll grow up eating healthy.

But what about the rest of you? Your kids are several years old, and you've already "ruined" them with chips, crackers, and cookies, and they completely refuse anything green or brown.

Take heart. Of course, you haven't really ruined them. You (like 99 percent of Americans) just never thought it mattered much, but our book has now opened your eyes to the truth. You have your work cut out for you, and throughout this book you will read countless useful tips to get your kids to eat healthy. You will become an expert in PR (Pantry Relations) and be able to successfully market your new shopping list to your family. (Be forewarned: Your husband may be the hardest sell.)

For now, we want you to realize one simple truth: Your kids may eat less during these months of transition. They'll whine, they'll grumble, they'll sneak out with Dad to grab fast food at every chance they get. But remember: No child in the United States has ever starved because their parents stopped buying junk. Perhaps the biggest barrier to these changes is a well-meaning mother who worries so much that her kids won't eat that she continues to feed them junk just so they'll grow. If that describes you, we ask you to trust us, and trust your children's bodies. They will eventually accept these changes. In fact, their hearts, brains, muscles, hormones, bones, skin, and immune systems will love you for it (even if their attitudes don't quite so quickly). They'll grow up without heart disease, diabetes, high blood pressure, cancer, and a whole host of chronic diseases. Maybe when they're in their seventies and are able to play tackle football with their grandchildren, they'll stop and finally realize, "Hey, I'm still active and healthy, and I have my mother to thank for it!"

Dr. Bob realized this one Mother's Day when all the kids were going around the dinner table saying one thing they were most thankful to their mom for:

I told her that I remember how much I hated eating healthy foods when I was growing up. I always grumbled. I whined that we never had anything white in the house (no white sugar, white bread, or white noodles). I told her how eternally grateful I am now that she fed us healthy foods. And I'm passing these same lessons on to my own kids. Her high standards of nutrition will affect many generations of Searses, and we have her to thank for it.

So take heart. Hang in there. Stand up for what you believe in. Say no to junk, and say yes to a long and healthy life for your entire family. We'll show you how.

Give your children the gift of health. Try this mental exercise. Imagine you have passed on, and your children are gathered for the reading of your last will and testament. (Stay with me — it has a happy ending.) After reading a list of all the stuff each child receives, the trustee reads the last line: "And to all my children I leave the gift of health." What a wonderful gift to give! Of course, you cannot bequeath good health to your children by writing it into your will. But you can give your children the gift of health by teaching them to enjoy healthy food. And you don't have to wait to do this — you can start right now.

3

Feed Your Family the Right Carbs

Let's clear up the carb confusion. There's a lot of misinformation about carbs floating around thanks to the recent fad for low-carb diets. First, carbs are not bad things. Kids need carbs to grow, think, and play. Like fuel for a moving car, carbs provide energy for active bodies and brains. In fact, just like adults, active and growing children need around 50 percent of their daily calories in the form of carbohydrates, and even more when they are very active. Yet kids need the good-for-you carbs, not the junky carbs that make them fat and sick.

FEED YOUR FAMILY A GOOD-CARB DIET, NOT A LOW-CARB DIET

What makes a carb the healthy kind of carb? Carbs are good or bad depending on how they behave in the body. A good-for-you carb makes the body and brain feel good and perform well. A bad-for-you (or junky) carb causes all kinds of havoc. One way to tell them apart is by the company they keep. A carb that comes packaged with ample protein and/or fiber (and sometimes healthy fat) is good for you. A junky carb stands alone. It's as simple as that.

Here's how we explain this to kids: "A good-for-you carb holds hands with two friends, Mr. Protein and Ms. Fiber. A good-for-you carb always plays with these two friends; it never plays alone. These two good friends, protein and fiber, make the healthy carbs behave well in the body. A junky carb has no friends. It plays alone."

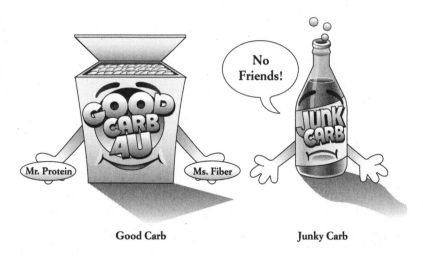

Good Carb   Junky Carb

Junky carbs are often known as empty calories because they don't come with any other nutrients your body needs, such as protein, fiber, or vitamins and minerals. For example, sodas and some sweetened beverages are just sugar water. Because junky carbs are not filling, soon after you eat them, your tummy feels empty, so you tend to overeat them.

Notice that all the healthy carbs have one thing in common: They spend little or no time being processed in a factory. Most come straight from nature, and nature makes few nutritional mistakes. Whole grains are ground into flour at a factory, but all of the grain, even the outer shell that provides the fiber, remains in

HEALTHY CARBS Contain Fiber and Protein	JUNKY CARBS Contain Little or No Fiber and Protein
• fruits • legumes, e.g., beans, peas, lentils • nut butters, e.g., peanut butter, almond butter • soy foods, e.g., tofu, soy drinks • veggies • whole grains, e.g., oatmeal, brown rice, whole wheat bread • yogurt, organic	• candy • cereals with fewer than 3 grams of protein and fiber per serving • chips • desserts and pastries • high-fructose corn syrup • sweetened beverages • white bread and pasta

the finished product. White flour goes through more processing stages. The outer bran is removed from the grain before it is made into flour, and (ironically) the flour then has to be enriched with various vitamins to make up for the ones lost when the bran was removed. Another way to look at it is, if it grows in nature, it's good for you; if it's factory made, it's suspect.

Also, you will notice that the healthy carbs on the list have at least one friend to hold hands with: fiber, protein, or fat. The junky carbs are on their own, or sometimes, as in packaged bakery goods, they hang out with fats that aren't good for you.

Carbs include various kinds of sugars, including table sugar. So, what about the sugar listed on package labels — is it healthy or not? Go back to our definition of a healthy carb: one that holds hands with two friends, namely protein and fiber. The way

> ### NUTSHELL
> ### "Healthy Food" –
> ### What Do You Call It?
> We use the terms "healthy" and "junky" when referring to carbs and fats. If your child equates "healthy" with "icky," try using "good carbs" or "grow carbs."

table sugar behaves in the body is the result of the company it keeps. Put a load of table sugar (also known as sucrose) or corn syrup in water, add artificial flavors, and you have a sweetened beverage that behaves badly in the body because the sugar is all by itself, with no nutritious friends to make it behave. Yet, to make it behave, put a bit of sugar with a bowl of whole-grain cereal and it behaves as a good carb because it is joined by fiber and protein. (To learn how to identify healthy and junky carbs on package labels, see Lessons in Label Reading, page 249.)

TAKE A CARB TRIP THROUGH THE BODY

Healthy carbs act like a time-release energy capsule in the body, delivering fuel to cells at a steady rate just when they need it. To appreciate how some carbs "behave" and other carbs "misbehave," let's follow them through the body. We'll make stops at all the systems and see how different the two kinds of carbs are.

Shaping young tastes. First stop is the taste buds, which detect sweetness. Sweet is the taste right on the tip of your tongue, so your first impression of a food tells you whether it's sweet or not. Infant tongues are especially programmed to enjoy sweetness because Mother's milk is sweet. Many healthy carbs are sweet — fruits and some veggies — yet not intensely. The fiber, and some protein, that they are packaged with mellows the sweet taste so it is pleasant and interesting.

Junky carbs — the kind where sugar stands alone, with no nutritious friends — tend to overwhelm the taste buds with sweetness. Sugar as it is found in nature — for example, in sugarcane, sweet corn, and sugar beets — is only mildly sweet until the fiber of the cane, corn, or beets is removed in the refining process. Concentrated sugar by the spoonful was never intended to hit our taste buds. But with repeated exposure to sugar in this form, we start to believe that this is what food is supposed to taste like. We crave overly sweetened foods and eat too much of them while shunning the more subtle flavors of natural food. Kids learn to prefer a sugary cupcake to an apple. The trouble starts, though, when their parents don't know how to say no and the occasional treat becomes a daily indulgence.

Filling young tummies. Next stop, the stomach. Good-for-you carbs leave the body feeling satisfied, not wanting more. The healthy fat, protein, and fiber that accompany healthy carbs come with a high-satiety index. We call them "fill-up foods." This means they fill you up and trigger the appestat, the communication network between the gut and the brain, to send a message that says, "I've eaten enough, and I'm satisfied."

Carbs that partner with fiber enjoy another appetite-curbing advantage. Because they take longer to chew and swallow than foods lacking fiber, high-fiber carbs are eaten and digested more slowly. You feel full without eating as much. Also, all that chewing sends increased amounts of saliva into the gut. Saliva is the body's own health juice. It

NUTSHELL
The healthier the carb, the more filling it is.

lubricates the lining of the intestinal tract so that food slides through better. And saliva contains enzymes that start to digest carbs as you chew, making less work for your stomach and intestines. Saliva also buffers the irritating effects of stomach acids.

The more saliva, the better the gut feeling. (For more on the good gut feeling, see page 15.)

The sugar rush hour. Finally, our last stop, the bloodstream. The lining of the gut is richly supplied with blood vessels. It is estimated that stretched out, the surface area of an adult intestine would match that of a football field. So as you can see, there is a lot of "playing surface" available to absorb nutrients from food.

Carbs enter the bloodstream in different ways. Healthy carbs are absorbed slowly. Their teammates — fat, fiber, and protein — keep them from rushing into the bloodstream too quickly. Fat, fiber, and protein all take longer to be broken down and digested than carbohydrates. They slow down the digestive process so that the food energy from the carbs enters the bloodstream slowly, over a longer period of time, instead of all at once. The cells of the body can then depend on a steady supply of energy — not too much, not too little.

HOW JUNKY CARBS MISBEHAVE IN THE BODY

Junky carbs are fast carbs. Because they have no friends to hold them back, they rush into the bloodstream quickly and overwhelm the energy delivery system. Then all sorts of mischief begins to take place that makes the body feel sick and tired rather than energized. Here's what can happen.

Junky carbs insult insulin. Junky carbs are a major contributor to the development of insulin-resistant diabetes. Here's how the body's sugar-using system can malfunction, causing blood sugar levels to soar.

The digestive system breaks carbohydrates down into the simple sugar glucose, which provides energy for all the cells of the body. Glucose gets to the cells via the bloodstream. To get inside the cells, glucose needs assistance from insulin, a hormone produced by the pancreas. On the surface of every cell are receptors that welcome insulin. When insulin from the blood parks itself in one of these receptors, it's like a button is pushed and a door opens to let glucose come into the cell. But when carbohydrates are digested too fast, there's a lot of glucose in the blood. The more glucose there is in the blood, the more insulin is released by the pancreas.

But there's a limit to how much glucose can get through the cell doors. Eventually the cells cry "Overload!" and the insulin is no longer able to activate the automatic buttons that open the doors and usher glucose into the cells. The cells resist what the insulin is telling them to do, and over time, Type 2 diabetes (also called insulin-resistant diabetes) can develop. If the diabetes is left untreated (the symptoms are not as obvious as in Type 1 diabetes), all that extra glucose circulating in the blood will do serious damage throughout the body. The body eventually pays a hefty price for the "fast living" of these fast carbs.

Junky carbs make you sick. Parents of frequently ill children often tell us, "You know, once we cleaned up his diet, he hasn't been sick as often." Excess junky carbs can depress the immune system. Besides causing excessive inflammation throughout the body (see Don't Raise an iBod, page 38), excess junky carbs suppress white blood cell function, the soldier cells that circulate throughout the body and kill invading germs. Drinking two and a half 12-ounce sodas can reduce the germ-killing ability of white blood cells by 40 percent. The effect can begin within fifteen minutes and can last for a few hours.

Junky carbs make you fat. We call healthy carbs "lean carbs," and junky carbs "fat carbs." Sedentary bodies may not be able to use all the sugar released into the bloodstream by the digestion of junky carbs. So, what happens to the excess sugar floating around in the bloodstream? It has to be stored somewhere. The body turns it into fat and deposits the fat in warehouses all over the body. These warehouses have a seemingly unlimited capacity. The more excess sugar the body needs to store, the bigger the warehouses get. Waistlines, arms, and thighs expand as the warehouses do; some children "fill out" way beyond what is healthy.

The problems that result are more critical than just needing to buy bigger jeans. Fat, especially fat deposited in the abdomen, around all the body's important organs, doesn't just sit there. It spews out all kinds of chemicals that increase a child's risk for diabetes, cancer, strokes, and cardiovascular disease. (Read more about the serious problems caused by excess abdominal fat on page 202.)

Consider the carbs in an apple. Because it has fiber in it, these carbs are slower to get into the bloodstream. (The fructose sugars in fruit and the galactose sugars in dairy first have to make a stop at the liver to be broken down into glucose before they can be released into the rest of the bloodstream, so they don't trigger insulin as much in the first place.) In a nutshell, "fat carbs" trigger the insulin cycle faster. "Lean carbs" don't trigger the insulin cycle as much, so they are less likely to be stored as fat. Also, because "lean carbs" are packaged with fiber, fat, or protein, you're less likely to overeat them than you are "fat carbs," which are not packaged with the *fill-up factor* of protein, fat, or fiber.

HOW JUNKY CARBS MISBEHAVE IN THE BRAIN

One day I was talking about carbs with nine-year-old Jacob in my office. I was telling Jacob how certain foods help him get better grades and pay attention better at school. After hearing my explanation, he said, "Dr. Bill, you mean there are smart foods and dumb foods?" Jacob was nutritionally correct.

Healthy carbs are smart foods. The brain depends on them. While the brain makes up around 2 percent of a child's total body weight, it utilizes around 50 percent of the carbs the child eats. The brain prefers healthy carbs because their slow and steady rate of digestion provides energy at a steady rate. In contrast, junky carbs flood the bloodstream and the brain with more sugar than it can handle. The excess sugar causes a problem. First, it stimulates the release of serotonin, a neurotransmitter that sedates the brain. This is one reason you should avoid feeding kids junky carbs at breakfast — those busy little brains need to be as alert as possible at school. (See the discussion of brainy breakfasts on page 188.)

Next, excess sugar makes the brain jittery: All that glucose in the bloodstream stimulates the pancreas to release a lot of insulin. The insulin mops up the glucose quickly, and blood sugar levels plunge. Suddenly the brain does not have enough fuel, and it crashes. Kids who are fed junky carbs for breakfast feel anxious and jittery by midmorning and can't concentrate on their schoolwork — they rebound from high to low blood sugar.

Unlike muscles, which store their own sugar supply to which they have continuous access, the brain doesn't store sugar. It must depend on a steady supply of sugar from the blood. This is why grazing on healthy carbs helps the brain work at peak efficiency. Frequent small meals of healthy carbs digested at a slow, steady rate provide just the right amount of sugar all the time. We suspect that the epidemic of learning disabilities in schoolchildren might be helped a great deal by eliminating "feeding disabilities" — brains functioning at less-than-optimal levels because of junky breakfasts.

Junky carbs stress out the brain. The ups and downs of blood sugar resulting from the too-fast digestion of junky carbs causes a child problems that go well beyond a fuel-deprived brain. Too much of the hormone insulin in the blood throws other hormones out of balance. When blood sugar plummets, the body sends out a survival signal: "I need more sugar, and fast!" This triggers the release of stress hormones, such as cortisol, from the adrenal glands. Cortisol tells the liver to release the sugar stored there, sending the blood sugar levels back up. Now the child has to cope with the high levels of stress hormones, which make him unsettled and unhappy. He pokes the kid next to him or talks to a classmate when he's supposed to be quietly working on his math. Soon he's in trouble with his teacher. Biochemical instability leads to emotional instability, which makes it hard for children to cope with their social and educational environments.

We think of a healthy breakfast as a "Happy Meal" and try never to choose an "Unhappy Meal."

CARBS AS "DRUGS"

Parents and teachers often forget that substances in food can alter behavior just as drugs do. Junky carbs can act like drugs, especially when you partner them with the caffeine, artificial flavors, and chemical colorings found in soft drinks and sweets. And, like many other mood-altering substances, junky carbs are addictive.

Carb-craving chemistry. Junky carbs affect brain biochemistry in ways similar to mood-changing drugs. Some children are especially sensitive to carb cravings and therefore to becoming addicted to junky carbs.

When carbs hit the brain, they trigger the release of serotonin. Serotonin in just the right amount provides a sense of contentment and relaxation. A number of antidepressant drugs, including Prozac and Zoloft, elevate mood by increasing the amount of serotonin floating around in the brain. Junk-carb addicts learn to associate happy feelings with eating carbs. So when stress levels go up or unhappiness strikes, they go looking for candy, cakes, cookies, ice cream — foods full of junky carbs (and other harmful things) that are digested quickly and produce a quick "hit" of serotonin. In time, the junk-carb craver comes to depend upon junky food to stay in a happy mood.

Carb cravings do serve a useful biochemical purpose. One carb-craving hormone called neuropeptide-Y (NPY) ensures that the brain gets enough sugar for energy. When blood sugar stores get too low to provide enough energy for the brain, NPY sends the signal "You need to eat." But the stress hormone cortisol also triggers the release of NPY, so stress leads to carb cravings. (Other effects of cortisol include the release of insulin, which not only heightens the carb cravings but also tells the body to store excess energy as fat.) It's a vicious cycle. The more junk carbs you eat, the more you crave.

HEALTHY CARBS VS. JUNKY CARBS: HOW THEY BEHAVE

Healthy Carbs	Junky Carbs
• fill you up, so you don't overeat	• leave you feeling hungry, so you eat more than you should
• help you feel energetic	• make you feel tired
• help your brain think clearly	• can cause fuzzy thinking
• help keep you from getting sick	• can make you sick by depressing your immunity
• help keep you lean	• can make you fat
	• leave you craving more

Many mothers notice that their children get squirrelly and restless after drinking a can of soda or eating sweets. As they come down from one sugar high, feeling hungry and stressed-out, they look for the carbs that will produce the next one. It's as if carb-sensitive kids are medicating themselves when they go on a carbohydrate binge.

REALLY JUNKY CARBS

There are junky carbs, and then there are *really* junky carbs. Take soda, for example. Sodas are made of a sweetener, carbonated water, and various substances, mostly artificial, that add flavor and color. They contain not one milligram of protein, fiber, or fat to slow down the digestion process. And they have no nutritional value whatsoever. Soda is a really junky carb, and some sodas are worse than others.

Nondiet sodas and juice drinks are sweetened with high-fructose corn syrup (HFCS), a carb that is not found in nature. (HFCS, the number one commercial sweetener, supplies nearly 10 percent of all calories consumed by Americans. This percentage is even higher for some children.) Because of the term "high fructose," the perception is that it is healthy. Some researchers believe that HFCS is even more unhealthy for humans than excess table sugar.

Martha notes: *Twenty-five years ago I thought the new high-fructose corn syrup was healthier than sugar, because I thought fructose was fruit. That tricked me into giving my children HFCS-sweetened drinks. Now I know better!*

HFCS is used by beverage companies and food processors because it is cheap to produce. While sucrose, or table sugar, is made from sugarcane or sugar beets, HFCS comes from corn, not fruit.* The corn crop is subsidized by the U.S. government, so there is always plenty of corn on the market, which makes HFCS cheaper to produce. It is the darling of the food industry because it's more stable in solution (i.e., dissolved in carbonated water to make soda) than table sugar. This means that HFCS-sweetened products have a longer shelf life than those made with sucrose, or table sugar. Also, table sugar loses some of its sweetness in the acidic environment of carbonated water.

Sucrose and HFCS appear to be similar, since they're both about 50 percent fructose and 50 percent glucose. (To be exact, HFCS-55 is 55 percent fructose and 42 percent glucose, with 3 percent other sugars, while natural sucrose is 50-50.) But there's a basic difference. Sucrose is a disaccharide, which means that the fructose and glucose are linked by a chemical bond that is broken down by an enzyme in the lining of the small intestines. In the case of HFCS, the fructose and glucose are free and un-bonded to each other. Does this matter? Corn syrup manufacturers claim that since HFCS has nearly the same 50-50 combination of glucose and fructose as table sugar, the body can't tell the difference and handles both kinds of sweeteners in the same way. Some nutrition researchers are not convinced of this.

Some researchers believe that HFCS increases blood fats (called triglycerides) more than the same amount of table sugar does. High triglyceride levels can lead to higher blood levels of LDL, the bad cholesterol, and to lower blood levels of HDL, the good cholesterol — a double whammy that increases the risk of cardiovascular disease. Imagine the insult to your child's arteries after eating a double cheeseburger and a supersize bottle of

---

* In the early '70s, researchers developed a process in which three enzymatic (chemical) reactions are used to convert cornstarch into HFCS. These enzymes break down the cornstarch into very small sugar molecules — exactly what we've been saying you should avoid.

HFCS-sweetened soda. Also, some researchers say that a diet high in HFCS can impair the body's ability to use minerals such as calcium and chromium — minerals that are involved in normal sugar and fat metabolism. In one study, the addition of HFCS to a high-fat meal increased the after-meal level of triglycerides. Another study showed that HFCS-sweetened soft drinks reduced blood levels of calcium and phosphorus, minerals needed for healthy bones.

In addition, some consumers are concerned about HFCS because it can come from corn that is a genetically modified organism (GMO). We agree with the opinion of Dr. Andrew Weil: "While food manufacturers view the development of HFCS as revolutionary, I consider it a crying shame. . . . I avoid foods with HFCS." Here's why we believe you should not feed your kids foods that list high-fructose corn syrup among the ingredients:

Can HFCS make you fat? Researchers studying the epidemic of childhood obesity believe that increased consumption of HFCS-sweetened beverages could be one of the causes. Between 1970 and 1974 the per capita annual average of HFCS consumption was only 1.5 pounds. By the year 2000, it had skyrocketed to 62.7 pounds. The rise in the incidence of childhood obesity parallels this increase in the consumption of HFCS-sweetened beverages. The correlation between the two does not prove that HFCS is a cause of childhood obesity, but it certainly suggests that we need to take a closer look at the effects of high-fructose corn syrup on kids' metabolism. There are several reasons for believing that HFCS is making kids fat.

First, corn syrup is guilty by association. It shows up (as sugar used to show up) mostly in junk foods and junk beverages. HFCS even shows up in otherwise healthy foods like yogurt. One easy shopping tip we pass on to parents in our pediatric practice is just to not buy any food containing high-fructose corn syrup. Following this one simple rule could eliminate as much as 90 percent of the junk food in your child's diet.

Another problem with HFCS is that it may not trigger the same feelings of fullness and satisfaction that regular sugar does. Table sugar is a low-satiety food, which means you eat more than is good for you before you feel satisfied. HFCS is even worse. Unlike other sugars, HFCS doesn't trigger the release of the hormone leptin, part of the body's natural food-volume regulation system, which sends out a signal when you've eaten enough. Studies also show that a large amount of fructose in the diet may increase the risk of developing insulin resistance. So, sweetened beverages have a triple fault: the type of sweetener they contain, the amount of sweetener, and the fact that the sweetener is not partnered with the appetite-satisfying nutrients fiber, protein, or fat. That's why some endocrinologists have dubbed HFCS-sweetened beverages "diabetes in a bottle."

A patient in our practice exhibited some erratic behavior during her early school years. We finally traced the cause to a sensitivity to corn syrup. Once her parents eliminated HFCS from her diet, while still allowing some sugar, her behavior became pleasant. During her late teen years, this metabolic quirk returned, and by age twenty she developed insulin resistance (early Type 2 diabetes), requiring medication to control her blood sugar. Her endocrinologist predicted she would need this medication for the rest of her life. This patient set out to disprove her doctor's prediction. Over the next few years she made all the changes we advise in this book. She has been free of insulin resistance and off medication for four years — thanks to getting on the right track to muster up her own internal medicine.

LOW-GLYCEMIC FOODS ARE GOOD FOR YOU

Perhaps you have heard the term "low-glycemic foods." The glycemic index (GI) is a laboratory measure of how quickly a carbohydrate is digested and how much it raises the blood sugar.

Some fruits, most vegetables, and most protein foods (meat, fish, dairy) have a low GI. They enter the bloodstream slowly, triggering a less-intense insulin response, resulting in steadier blood-sugar levels. Processed foods and sweetened beverages (fiberless and proteinless foods) have a high GI. They rush into the bloodstream quickly and jolt the body into producing insulin. Blood sugar levels rise and fall like a roller coaster, stressing mind and body. A carb with a low GI is a slow carb, and one with a high GI is a fast carb. You can look up a food's GI in books on nutrition or on the Internet, but it's easier to remember this general principle: Healthy carbs — those packaged with fiber, protein, or fat — tend to have a low GI, and junky carbs — the ones that go it alone — tend to be high-GI carbs. For example, white bread has a higher GI than whole wheat bread.

TWELVE TIPS TO CURB YOUR CHILD'S CARB CRAVINGS

Do you and your kids have a hard time controlling your carb cravings? Can you eat just one cookie, or do you need half a dozen? Do your children crave soda and sweetened sports beverages? You are not alone. For many people, because eating sweets triggers an increase in levels of serotonin, the body and brain come to depend on carbs for a sense of well-being. When the serotonin level dips, carb cravers use soda or sweets to boost their mood again. Or they crave a high-carbohydrate breakfast after using up their carbohydrate stores during many hours of sleep. (A high-carb breakfast is okay, but make sure it's a healthy-carb breakfast and includes some protein!) In contrast, fat cravings tend to be highest in the evening, when the body needs to store fat for the overnight fast.

Kids like carbs, and they always will. Your job is to get them to crave healthy carbs and stay away from the junky ones. Here are some time-tested tips:

1. Shape tastes in infancy. Babies are born with a sweet tooth, so you need to shape those little tastes in a healthy-carb direction right from the start. Here's how:

- Breastfeed for as long as possible.
- Make your own baby food from fresh fruits and vegetables.
- Use infant and toddler foods with no added sweeteners.
- Dilute juices (25 percent juice to 75 percent water).
- Avoid giving babies sugar- or corn syrup–sweetened beverages and artificial sweeteners.

Parents, don't be nutritional wimps. A mother in our practice offered this excuse: "My child will only eat yogurt sweetened with corn syrup." Who's in charge here? Instead of shaping your child's tastes toward unreal sweeteners, add fruit, like blueberries, to plain yogurt.

2. Always partner carbs with protein and fiber. To blunt the blood sugar highs and lows of a high-carb meal, be sure that meals — and snacks — have adequate protein and fiber. Numbers may vary slightly depending on the age of the child, but as a general guide:

- For meals, shoot for the five-plus-five rule: Each carb meal should contain at least 5 grams of protein and 5 grams of fiber.

- For snacks, shoot for three-plus-three rule. Each carb snack should contain at least 3 grams of protein and 3 grams of fiber.

(For snack and meal recipes that partner carbs with plenty of protein and fiber, see chapter 12.)

3. Red-light sweetened beverages. Above all, limit your child's liquid carbs — those sweetened beverages that are simply liquid candy, containing all carbs and no protein and fiber. These include sodas, sports drinks, juice drinks, and anything else whose main ingredients are water plus sugar or corn syrup. Don't stock them in your pantry, and don't even buy them. If you buy junk carbs, your children will assume it's okay for them to eat and drink them. If children are offered an occasional sweetened beverage as a sweet treat, be sure they drink it with a meal.

NUTSHELL

To avoid the hormonal havoc that follows a sugar rush, don't drink sweetened beverages by themselves.

4. Have them graze on frequent mini-meals. Grazing steadies the blood sugar level. See chapter 6 for why grazing is good for kids.

5. Crave-proof your kitchen. If the junky carbs are in your kitchen, how can you expect your child not to want them? Banish the junky carbs and fill your cabinets and refrigerator with healthy-carb snacks, carbs that are packaged naturally with protein and fiber. Keep water bottles handy so that thirsty kids learn to drink no-carb water rather than high-carb beverages. (For healthy-carb snack suggestions, see page 167.) Cute water bottles may sound frivolous, especially if they are not in your budget, but if they help make water look appealing to your kids, they're worth it.

Dr. Bob shares how he "waters" his own kids:

In our kitchen we keep a water dispenser (with large bottles delivered to our house). The kids love getting their own water and watching the bubbles gurgle up in the bottle. The nozzle is kid proof, so toddlers can't drain water all over the floor. I think our kids drink a lot more water this way than if they had to ask us for help getting it out of the kitchen faucet.

6. Banish junky-carb cues. Carb cravers are notoriously susceptible to carb cues that trigger their cravings, such as TV ads and fast-food restaurants. The solution? Less TV and fewer restaurant meals. Out of sight is out of mind.

7. Tell them to move rather than eat. Kids who are bored or stressed are likely to crave carbs. Physical activity will take care of the craving and the stress or boredom. Tell your children, "When you feel the urge to eat, get up and run instead." Send kids outside to shoot baskets, kick the soccer ball around, turn cartwheels on the lawn, or just race around the park.

Learning to work off cravings and mood upsets with physical activity is a valuable tool for children, and a habit that will benefit them for the rest of their lives. Exercise stimulates the release of feel-good hormones, just as sugar does, and it's good for the body! Research has shown that the calm feeling that follows a workout decreases the appetite, especially carb cravings. In fact, an interesting study showed that following a brisk walk, carb cravers had a reduced urge to snack on sugary foods.

8. Serve them a brainy breakfast. See page 188 for a discussion of how a healthy-carb breakfast can lessen a child's craving for junky carbs throughout the day, and page 191 for examples of brainy breakfasts.

9. Offer healthy snacks and control portions. Carb cravings help to make kids obese, and in turn, obesity perpetuates their cravings for carbs. Break the cycle by offering kids lean meals and lean snacks. Fruit and nuts are sweet and crunchy alternatives to cookies, chips, and crackers. They offer healthy carbs and other valuable nutrients. Nuts offer protein and healthy fats as well. When it's time for the occasional treat, give your child a couple of cookies rather than handing him the whole box. Never let your child eat out of a container. He won't know when to stop. (See chapter 9, Raise a Lean Family.)

10. Offer sweet substitutes. In trying to raise a sugar-free kid, you can satisfy a sweet tooth without serving foods that contain a lot of sugar or corn syrup sweeteners. Try these strategies:

- *Offer a hot sip.* For adults, sipping a hot beverage is a time-tested way to suppress hunger pangs. Fruit-flavored herbal teas offer flavor without carbs and calories. Some people enjoy a squirt of lemon juice in hot water for a calming, crave-easing treat. Even if your child is not yet a fan of warm drinks in mugs (with the exception of hot chocolate), make her aware of these alternatives by setting an example. Your little carb-craver will carry this information into her teenage and adult years and use it to help her stay on the right track.

- *Offer cinnamon.* Recent research has shown that this sweet-tasting spice makes insulin work more efficiently to stabilize blood sugar levels. As an added perk, it even reduces cholesterol levels and other artery-clogging fats in the blood. Sprinkle a teaspoon of cinnamon on cereal, oatmeal, or in a smoothie to heighten the sweet and healthy taste. (Note: This doesn't mean that Cinnabons, with their junk sugar and bad carbs, are good for you!) See Spice Up Your Child's Eating, page 207, to learn how spicy foods curb cravings and overeating.

- *Try fruit toppings.* Unsweetened fruit is a tasty way to sweeten yogurt or top pancakes and waffles. Our family favorite is blueberries. Mix 2 tablespoons of fresh or thawed frozen blueberries into cereal, oatmeal, or plain yogurt. Or try yogurt and ripe bananas on your morning waffle. Dr. Jim's family likes to mash organic strawberries with a fork. This makes a tasty topping on waffles or pancakes. Try whole-grain pancakes or waffles, or half whole-grain.

- *Try xylose.* Xylose (commercial name Xylitol) is a naturally occurring carbohydrate found in many fruits and vegetables, particularly plums, raspberries, and cauliflower. It is just as sweet as sucrose (table sugar), yet it has some molecular quirks that could make it a healthier carbohydrate. Xylose has 40 percent fewer calories. Unlike sucrose, xylose is absorbed slowly and incompletely through the small intestine into the blood; and once absorbed, it is metabolized independent of insulin. This metabolic quirk keeps it from triggering the roller-coaster effect of blood sugar swings that you get with sucrose. Xylose also inhibits the ability of bacteria to adhere to the teeth, reducing the production of acids that dissolve tooth enamel and lead to tooth decay, making it a less worrisome sweetener for the sweet tooth and a favorite ingredient in chewing gums. Yet, these apparent perks are not a license to overdose on xylose. Because it is not absorbed into the bloodstream as quickly as sucrose and may remain in the intestines longer, eating too much xylose too fast (more than the same amount of table sugar) can result in uncomfortable gas and diarrhea.

11. Abolish artificial sweeteners. We advise you not to give your child any food that contains an artificial sweetener, such as aspartame. Although aspartame contains 4 calories per teaspoon compared with 16 calories per teaspoon for table sugar, saving a mere 12 calories isn't worth the potential risks associated with ingesting chemicals. When we surveyed the research on the safety of artificial sweeteners, we saw a lot of controversial findings. The

HONEY, I SWEETENED THE KIDS!

Many parents ask, "Is honey better than sugar?" Some may argue with us, but we believe honey is nutritionally superior to ordinary table sugar — though only slightly so. Both table sugar and honey are made up of glucose and fructose, but honey enjoys a slightly lower glycemic index, meaning it does not raise the blood sugar as quickly as table sugar does. The fact that honey has a bit lower GI than table sugar leads us to conclude it must behave biochemically better in the body, even if the difference is slight. Consider these unique features of honey that give it a slight edge over sugar:

- Honey is one of the few sweeteners in nature that can be eaten without processing.
- Honey contains very small amounts of vitamins, minerals, and antioxidants not found in table sugar.
- Honey has some antibacterial, anti-inflammatory, and antiseptic properties. The less processed the honey, the greater its medicinal value.

U.S. Food and Drug Administration gives aspartame and other artificial sweeteners on the market the status of "generally regarded as safe" (GRAS). Don't you wonder what they mean by "generally"? Should you feed your kids chemicals that are "generally" safe? We believe that any chemically manufactured sweetener is suspect, especially for growing children, who are too precious to be experimented on. Besides, artificially sweetened beverages and snack foods won't curb your child's carb cravings or teach your kids to appreciate the healthy foods that are good for them. Serving your kids fake sweets only reinforces their desire for factory-made foods. We believe it's better to just leave these foods out of your family's diet (and out of your house).

Splenda is the trade name for sucralose, an artificial sweetener

Even though honey may enjoy a slight advantage over table sugar, it's the company honey keeps that labels it healthy or junky. Accompanied by protein, fiber, and fat (as in a whole-grain muffin), honey qualifies as a healthy carb. Spread on white bread, all by itself, it's a carb you'd do better to avoid.

Here are a few precautions about honey:

- Don't give honey to infants under one year. Honey can carry botulism spores, which can cause serious illness, or even death, in young infants. These spores are not a danger to children who are older than one year of age.
- Avoid dipping pacifiers in honey. The sticky stuff can cause tooth decay.
- When substituting honey for sugar in recipes, use less honey than you would sugar. Honey gives you more sweetness per tablespoon than sugar does.

used in thousands of processed foods. The manufacturers claim that Splenda is natural because it's made from sugar. They also claim that Splenda is a no-calorie sweetener, since, they claim, the body doesn't digest or metabolize it. Splenda promises the sweet taste of sugar without the calories or metabolic effects of digesting carbs. Sound too good to be true? We think so. We believe there are many reasons to be concerned about the safety of Splenda, especially for children.

- *How it's made.* Splenda starts out as sugar, but the manufacturing process adds three chlorine atoms to the sugar molecule. This changes the molecule into a chlorocarbon that goes by the name "4,1',6'-trichlorogalactosucrose" and tastes sweeter than table sugar. Chlorocarbons are not known for doing healthy things for the body.

- *How it's metabolized.* If Splenda isn't absorbed by the body, as the manufacturers claim, why worry about its safety? Research reports in the Federal Register, the official publication of the U.S. Food and Drug Administration, state that 20 to 30 percent of ingested Splenda *is* metabolized by human subjects. Most of the studies about how the body uses Splenda were performed in animals such as mice, rats, rabbits, and dogs, which metabolize the substance differently from humans. There were wide variations in sucralose metabolism among these animals and also individual variations within each species and among the human subjects. So the claim that Splenda is not absorbed by the body is not true.

- *How it may affect children.* There are no studies of the long-term effects of Splenda on humans — adults or children. The manufacturer claims that Splenda is okay, even for kids with Type 1 or Type 2 diabetes, but again, there are no long-term studies. Some research shows slower weight gain in growing animals that have been fed Splenda. Is it safe to feed your children a chemical that could affect their normal growth?

- *How the gut feels about Splenda.* Even if most of the Splenda is not absorbed, as the manufacturer claims, it still hangs around in the gut for many hours. How does the gut feel about that? Does Splenda alter the normal flora of the gut, the beneficial bacteria that help digest your food and keep your intestines healthy? We don't know. We couldn't find any studies that address this issue.

- *How it shapes tastes.* Remember that you are trying to shape your child's tastes to prefer the natural sweetness of foods like fruits and some vegetables. Do you really want your children to experience food that is even sweeter than sugar? Aren't you a little suspicious of a packaged food that needs an artificial sweetener to make it flavorful and appealing?

Based on what we've read, we believe that sucralose and aspartame have not been proven safe for anyone, and especially not for children. With factory-made sweeteners we believe that the best rule is: When in doubt, leave it out. We advise you to keep foods made with artificial sweeteners away from your kids. (See AskDrSears.com/updates for the latest information on the artificial sweetener controversy and other sugar substitutes.)

12. Limit added "sugar." Surprising amounts of sugar lurk in many store-bought processed foods such as ketchup, spaghetti sauce, barbecue sauce, baked beans, and even soup. While a teaspoon or so of sugar (4–5 grams) in an otherwise healthy whole-grain cereal (one with at least 5 grams of protein and 3 grams of fiber) is fine for kids (though a tablespoon of fruit is a healthier sweetener), too much added sugar can turn a healthy food into oversweetened, unhealthy junk. Fruit-flavored yogurt is a leading example. Compare the nutrition information on plain yogurt with one flavored with fruit. There is less protein but there are a lot more carbs and a lot more calories in the flavored variety, and all of those extra carbs are fast carbs from sugar or corn syrup sweeteners. The carbs in plain yogurt come from milk (lactose), and the protein (and in some, fat) in the yogurt slows their absorption.

The World Health Organization (WHO) recommends limiting added sugars in the diet to 6 teaspoons per 1,000 calories consumed per day. That's less sugar than you'll find in one 12-ounce serving of soda. It is nearly impossible for parents to determine how much sugar has been added to processed foods. The sugars line on the Nutrition Facts label gives the amount of sugar per serving, but it does not differentiate between sugar that naturally occurs in a food and added sugar. In plain yogurt, the amount of sugar listed on the label is nearly equal to the amount of total carbs. Plain yogurt has no added sugar, yet the natural sugar lactose gets the same treatment on the label as table sugar or high-fructose corn syrup. To get a sense of how much sweetener has been added to a food, be sure to check the ingredients list as well as the nutrition information. Ingredients are listed from greatest amounts to least. If sugar or corn syrup appears near the top of the list, you may want to avoid this food.

The first change in getting your family on the right track is to change your carbs. In the next chapter you will learn why and how to change your fats.

4

Feed Your Family a Right-Fat Diet

One day, following a talk Dr. Bill gave at Harvard Medical School on kids' nutrition, a doctor in the audience asked, "What do you consider the number-one nutritional deficiency in American families?" Dr. Bill surprised the audience by answering, "In my opinion, it's healthy fats."

Anyone who knows anything about what Americans eat knows that most of us eat too much fat. So it may surprise you to hear that you and your children need to eat *more* fat — that is, more of certain kinds of fat. Just as with carbs, there are good-for-you fats and bad-for-you fats, fats you should eat more of and fats to avoid. Read this chapter to learn more about what kinds of fats to eat and which foods contain them.

WHY KIDS NEED FATS

Growing children need fat in their diet. Fat is a component of many important parts of the body and of the substances that make the body work well. Kids need to have the right kinds of fat in their diets so that their bodies can build healthy tissue and operate at an optimal level. Here's why children need healthy fats:

Fats build the brain. The brain is 60 percent fat. The structural components of cell membranes throughout the body are made of fat, and having the right kinds of fats available to form these membranes is especially important in the brain. Fats build myelin, the fatty sheath that insulates nerves, like insulation on electrical wires. This insulation makes it possible for messages to travel efficiently throughout the brain and the body.

Fats help make hormones. Fats are structural components of some of the most important substances in the body, including sex hormones and prostaglandins, substances that regulate many functions in the body.

Fats build healthy skin. Fat under the skin keeps you from getting cold. It also gives the skin a smooth, nice-looking texture. We have found in our medical practice that one of the main clues that children are not getting enough healthy fats in their diet is scaly, dry skin.

Fats help the body use important vitamins. Fats in foods help the intestines absorb vitamins A, D, E, and K.

Fats protect and cushion the organs. Many vital organs, including the kidneys, heart, and intestines, are protected from injury by a cushion of fat.

Fats provide energy. Body fat stores energy. When the body runs out of fuel from a meal or snack and its small amount of stored carbs, it dips into its reserves and burns fat to keep you going.

Fats add to the pleasure of eating. Fats give foods an appealing texture and flavor. Fats carry more flavor than carbs and protein. They also give food a smooth and silky feeling in the mouth. Vegetables sautéed in a bit of olive oil have a more intense flavor and a silkier texture than steamed vegetables.

Fats are filling. Fats in food help you feel satisfied. Even though gram for gram, fats have twice as many calories as carbs, fats may actually help you eat fewer calories. Fats trigger the release of a satiety hormone called cholecystokinin, or CCK, in the stomach, which tells the brain you've eaten enough. Fats in a meal or snack also slow the entry of carbs into the bloodstream, so food is digested slowly and a feeling of fullness lasts longer than it would if low-fiber, low-protein carbs were eaten by themselves. Try this experiment. At snacktime, spread 2 tablespoons of peanut butter on slices of apple and enjoy. You've eaten approximately 230 calories. Notice how satisfied you feel and for how long. The next day try a different 230-calorie snack, but one with little or no fat, such as a large serving of fruit juice. You'll probably feel hungry again soon and want to eat more. The right amount of healthy fat is good for the body (though, as you will learn in chapter 9, it is possible to eat too much of a good thing).

THE BEST FATS FOR YOUR FAMILY

Not all fats are created equal. The standard American diet (SAD) has a double fat fault — too much of the wrong fats and too little of the right ones. Most American families eat excessive amounts of fats that come from animals and food factories and not enough fats from plants and fish. Healthy fats such as olive oil are liquid at room temperature. They flow. Unhealthy fats are made of molecules that clump together at room temperature, such as the solid

COLOR CODING FAT-CONTAINING FOODS

To get the right amount of the right kinds of fats in your family's diet, you need to serve more healthy fats and fewer unhealthy fats. Here's the traffic-light system applied to fats. *Green* means "go for it, eat lots!" These are "anytime" foods. *Yellow* means "slow down, okay to eat, but not too much." These are "sometimes" foods. *Red* means "stop, don't eat these foods!" These are "no time" foods.

Green-Light Foods		Yellow-Light Foods
avocados	olive oil	butter
eggs*	olives	canola oil
flaxseed oil	seafood, especially wild salmon	chocolate, dark
hummus		cocoa butter
meat, lean, and poultry, skinless†	seeds, e.g., sunflower, pumpkin	coconut oil
nut butters, e.g., peanut butter, almond butter	soy foods, e.g., tofu, soy drinks	corn oil
		ice cream
nuts	wheat germ	palm kernel oil

fat in an uncooked steak or the glob of vegetable shortening in the can on the supermarket shelf.

The best fats for your family are:

- avocado
- flaxseed oil
- nut butters, e.g., peanut butter, almond butter
- nuts, especially walnuts, almonds
- olive oil

Yellow-Light Foods		Red-Light Foods
safflower oil	bacon	partially hydrogenated oils
sunflower oil	chicken, fried	
	cottonseed oil	sausage
	hamburgers (fatty), hot dogs, and some lunch meats	trans fats
		vegetable shortening made from partially hydrogenated oils
	lard	

* We give egg yolks a green-light rating for kids but a yellow-light rating for some adults. Kids don't overeat eggs. Adults who have high levels of fat (triglycerides and cholesterol) in their bloodstream should eat egg yolks in moderation. Egg yolks are high in saturated fats and cholesterol, and, unlike seafood, their omega-fatty-acid profile can be pro-inflammatory, a concept you will learn more about on page 203.

† We give lean meat and skinless poultry a green-light rating for children because, unlike adults, children rarely overeat these foods.

- seafood, especially wild salmon
- seeds, e.g., flax, sesame, sunflower, pumpkin

The healthiest fats, those found in seafood and plants and known as polyunsaturated and monounsaturated fats, contribute to cardiovascular health because their fat molecules are curved in such a way that they flow better through the arteries. Heart-unhealthy fats are saturated fats (so-called because all the available receptor sites on the fat molecule are saturated with hydrogen atoms). These are the types of fats found in meat and other animal products. Their flat molecules pile up like pancakes and stick together, clogging the arteries. While the tissues of the body do need some saturated fats to grow optimally, the liver makes all the saturated fats the body needs. Unlike the omega fats in fish, which are called essential fats because, since the body can't make them, it's essential that you get them from foods, saturated fats don't need to be consumed. The body grows optimally with just the amount of saturated fats that the liver makes. Because a diet completely free of saturated fats is nearly impossible, and unnecessary, the American Heart Association recommends that persons of all ages limit their saturated fats to no more than 7 percent of the total daily calories, or approximately one-third of the total fat consumed. We believe less than this amount is best for optimal health.

THE WORST FATS FOR YOUR FAMILY

Why are we suddenly seeing "no trans fats" touted on food packaging? After decades of research exposed these factory-made fats as the worst kinds of fats, as of January 2006, manufacturers are now required to list the number of grams of trans fats on the Nutrition Facts label. Here's what parents should know about what trans fats are and why they're harmful to children's health.

Trans fats are so-called because a chemical process called hydrogenation transports hydrogen atoms from one side of the fat molecule to the other. Trans fats are artificially formed when food factories bubble hydrogen gas into vegetable oil, a process called partial hydrogenation. Chemically changing the fats in oils such as corn oil or soybean oil has economic advantages for food processors. It helps the oil withstand higher heat, making it a plus for deep-frying, and trans fats don't spoil as fast as the nonhydrogenated oils, so they give products a longer shelf life. While trans fats may lengthen the shelf life of foods, they certainly can shorten the life of growing bodies. Here's how.

NUTSHELL

Teach your children to avoid foods whose labels carry the bad words "trans fats" and "partially hydrogenated oils."

In chapter 7 on feeding growing brains, you'll learn why a healthy cell, especially a brain cell, needs to have a flexible membrane in order to grow and function properly. On each cell membrane reside millions of microscopic "parking spots" called receptor sites. Healthy fats, especially the omega-3 fats mentioned below, enter these reserved parking spots and contribute to the health of the cell membrane.

However, when trans fats fill up the parking spots reserved for the healthy fats, causing the cell membrane to become more rigid (due to the trans fat's molecular structure), they interfere with the cell membrane's growth and function. Besides causing mischief at the cellular level, diets high in trans fats do the following:

- raise LDL (bad cholesterol) in the blood and lower HDL (good cholesterol)
- decrease immunity
- interfere with nerve-cell function
- increase cardiovascular disease
- increase the risk of many cancers, especially colon cancer
- increase the incidence of Type 2 diabetes

Trans fats not only lead to obesity but, because of some biochemical quirk, also cause an increase in abdominal fat, which increases the risk of just about every disease.

To avoid feeding your family trans fats, be sure to read food labels. When dining out, inquire whether the food is fried in trans fats and if the salad dressings contain these harmful oils. If your server doesn't know, take your own salad dressing along, and don't order fried food anyway.

Parents and pediatricians often underestimate how well children can understand nutritional issues. Here's an example. One day I (Dr. Bill) was explaining the concept of healthy fats and unhealthy fats to one of my patients, Jacob, a "pure kid" from a nutrition-savvy family. After the checkup, I asked Jacob to write me a letter about what he had learned about hydrogenated fats and how this knowledge might affect his food choices. Here's what nine-year-old Jacob wrote:

> *Hydrogenated fats are bad fats. They inject foods with hydrogen so they can sit on the shelves. Then in a few years you can say, "Look, it's the doughnuts we got three years ago! They look as good as new." Hydrogenated fats clog up your arteries. My grandpa had this sort of problem. He died when he was fifty-five years old, before I was born. It's good to have goods last a long time, but how long your body lasts is a lot more important than how long your food lasts. I wish I had my grandpa.*

Jacob gets it!

FEED YOUR FAMILY MORE FISH

One kind of fat, the group known as omega-3 fatty acids, is especially good for you. Because your body cannot manufacture these fatty acids by itself, it's essential that you eat them. Omega-3 fatty acids play an important role in the body in maintaining the health of the cardiovascular system and the brain.

NUTSHELL
Feed your family more fat that comes from seafood and plants and less fat that comes from animals.

Fish fats are the healthiest fats, especially for growing bodies and brains, because they contain large amounts of omega-3 fatty acids. The greatest amounts of omega-3 fats are found in fish that swim in cold water — salmon, sardines, tuna, and trout. Population studies have shown that cultures that eat a lot of fish have a lower incidence of just about every illness, especially inflammatory disorders ("-itis" illnesses), such as gingivitis, colitis, dermatitis, and arthritis. Omega-3 oils can also improve lung function in children with asthma and in adults with chronic pulmonary disease.

Eat fish, be happy. The standard American diet (SAD) can make you sad. Neuroscientists suspect that increasing rates of depression in America, especially among children, may be related to a national diet that contains too many unhealthy fats and too few healthy ones. Consider the famous salmon study. Researchers divided depressed persons into two groups. One group was treated with a standard antidepressant medicine, and the other group was treated with a daily "dose" of salmon. At the end of the study, the salmon eaters experienced less depression than the persons treated with medication. The fish eaters were happier! (See page 173 for more about fish as a brain food.)

NUTSHELL
A serving of salmon a day helps keep depression away.

Eat fish, have a healthy heart. There are four things your child needs in order to have a healthy cardiovascular system (and that you need, too, to ensure you're likely to live long enough to walk your daughters down the aisle):

- The heartbeat should be regular.
- The lining of the arteries should be smooth so that plaque doesn't build up.

- The blood should be thin enough that it doesn't clot too easily and clog the arteries.
- The arterial wall must be flexible — no hardening of the arteries.

Cardiologists often prescribe medicines to help these good things happen. Yet all four of these heart-healthy effects can be helped by one "pill" — fish oil.

Seafood is good for your heart and your arteries, so it protects you from cardiovascular disease. The medical truism "You're only as healthy as your arteries" used to be what every practitioner of geriatrics advised senior citizens. Since the recent finding that coronary artery disease is occurring at a younger and younger age, this advice has also become a favorite of pediatricians. Studies reveal that over 70 percent of twelve-year-olds already show the beginning stages of hardening of the arteries. The

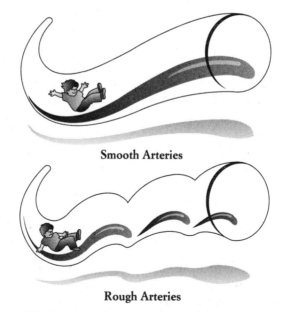

Smooth Arteries

Rough Arteries

Which arteries do you want your child to have?

heart-healthy omega-3 oils in seafood protect arteries from inflammation. High blood pressure, nicotine, diabetes, and many other things can cause the lining of the arteries to become inflamed. Inflammation promotes the buildup of fatty streaks called plaque in the arteries, rough spots where platelets from the blood and other kinds of gunk can accumulate and block the free flow of blood to the heart and brain. Eventually, the blockage can cause a heart attack or a stroke.

Doctors often suggest that patients at risk for cardiovascular disease take a small dose of aspirin every day to help prevent inflammation in the lining of the arteries and keep the blood from clotting too fast. Omega 3's have anti-inflammatory and anticoagulant properties that work in much the same way as aspirin does but without the potential side effects of intestinal irritation. You could think of heart-healthy oils such as fish oil as liquid aspirin. Simply put, omega 3's help keep the lining of the arteries smooth like Teflon, so that nothing can stick to them. Inflammation makes the lining of the arteries rough and sticky like Velcro. Omega-3 oils also help to lower blood cholesterol and blood pressure. Omega-3 oils even help regulate the heartbeat.

Eat fish, lower your risk of cancer. Population studies have shown that people who eat fatty fish, such as wild salmon, two times a week have a much lower rate of many cancers than people who eat less than this amount. Just as omega-3 oils help to repair damaged arteries, they may also inhibit the growth of malignant cells, preventing the growth of tumors.

Eat fish, prevent diabetes. Healthy fats like omega 3's help to stabilize blood sugar and thus lower the risk of Type 2, insulin-resistant diabetes. Pediatricians are increasingly concerned that younger and younger kids are developing Type 2 diabetes, thanks to diets high in processed carbs and low in healthy fats.

SAFE SEAFOOD

When you "go fishing" at the supermarket for healthy fats for your family, be sure you catch safe seafood. Pregnant and breastfeeding women need to be especially vigilant about eating safe seafood. Fish that come from contaminated waters contain chemicals that are potentially harmful. However, with the growing body of research validating the health benefits of seafood, doctors believe that many people are unnecessarily shying away from seafood because of the perceived risks. As long as you follow the safety precautions we mention below, the general medical opinion is that the health benefits of seafood far outweigh the risks.

Safest salmon. The safest kind of fish and the one that contains the healthiest omega-3 oils is wild Alaskan salmon. This is our top pick for safe and healthy seafood. Wild salmon has been found to contain fewer contaminants than farmed salmon, which tend to contain higher levels of PCBs, carcinogenic chemicals from environmental pollution. However, health experts believe that the health benefits of eating farmed salmon far outweigh any potential health risk from environmental contaminants. We agree. Still, it's good to know where your seafood comes from. Most canned salmon comes from wild fish. If the label says "Alaskan salmon," it must be wild, since fish farming is illegal in Alaska. "Atlantic salmon," which is the usual type served in restaurants, is nearly always farmed salmon. Supermarkets may not always label their seafood as "wild" or "farmed," so you might have to ask. For resources on where to buy safe and nutritious seafood, see www.AskDrSears.com/seafood.

Safest fish. Commonly eaten fish that are low in mercury include Alaskan salmon, shrimp, canned light tuna (lower than albacore), pollock (used in most fish sticks), catfish, Pacific cod, haddock, trout, Pacific halibut, and tilapia.

Risky fish. Avoid eating fish that consume large fish, like shark, swordfish, king mackerel, and tilefish, because they contain very high levels of mercury, which is toxic to growing bodies and brains. It's especially important for pregnant and breastfeeding women and growing children to avoid these fish. During the writing of this book, the mother of a family in our practice reported increasing fatigue, weakness, and muscle twitching and that her two children were developing symptoms of learning disabilities. We suspected that the cause of these problems was high levels of mercury in the shark and swordfish the family was frequently consuming. Testing revealed elevated mercury levels. After they avoided the offending fish for a few months, their symptoms disappeared.

Avoid eating fish that have been caught in lakes and rivers that are known to be polluted with environmental contaminants. For an update on safe seafood, call the U.S. Food and Drug Administration's Food Information Line toll free at 1-888-SAFEFOOD or visit the FDA's Food Safety website, www.cfsan.fda.gov/seafood1.html. You can get mercury information at the EPA's mercury website, www.epa.gov/mercury.

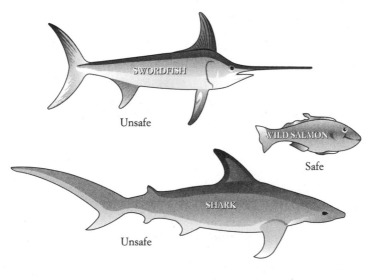

SWORDFISH
Unsafe

WILD SALMON
Safe

SHARK
Unsafe

SALMON VS. SIRLOIN

Let's follow a salmon fillet and a sirloin steak through your child's bloodstream and notice the immediate difference between a healthy fat and an unhealthy fat. When the omega-3 oils in the salmon enter the bloodstream, they do good things, such as open up the blood vessels and help more blood flow to growing organs. When the fats from a marbled sirloin enter the bloodstream, bad things happen, a risky change called "postprandial lipemia." Artery-clotting fats, such as triglycerides, build up inside the arteries. The inflammatory fat in the sirloin roughens the lining of the arteries and causes platelets to stick together (as a blood clot). To make matters worse, the coronary arteries and the arteries in the brain go into spasm and become narrower, which further slows the blood flow. You guessed it: After the sirloin meal, the brain and heart are set up for a stroke or heart attack. In adults we call this scenario the "Steakhouse Syndrome." In children, steak after steak gradually causes arteries to get too old and too clogged too fast. Studies show that a lesser arterial reaction occurs after we eat lean wild game that consumed healthy food and ran around all day than with sirloin from a steer that sat around in a fattening pen and ate junk food all day.

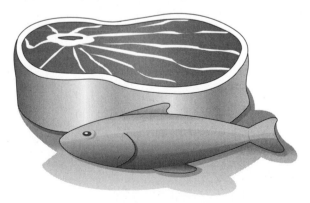

Eat fish, stay young. As we described above, omega 3's form the structural components of brain cells. As people age, cell membranes, like joints, become stiffer. Omega 3's help cell membranes throughout the body, including the brain, retain their flexibility, so the cells behave more like cells in a younger body. Studies have shown that senior citizens with higher blood levels of the brain-building fat docosahexaenoic acid (DHA) are less likely to show deterioration of brain function. A diet rich in omega-3 oils is now part of the "Maintain Your Brain" consumer education campaign promoted by the Alzheimer's Association. (See www.alz.org.)

Eat fish, stay lean. The same metabolic perk that causes a diet rich in omega 3's to decrease the risk of diabetes also helps keep the body lean. Omega 3's could rightly be called "lean fat."

For more on the health benefits of seafood, see Eat Fish, Be Smart, page 171. For fish-fixing tips, see our recipes on pages 309 and 313–316.

SCIENCE SAYS: SEAFOOD IS HEALTH FOOD!

Here's a summary of what current research says about the health benefits of seafood. People who eat more omega 3–containing fish (especially cold-water fish such as salmon) enjoy:

- healthier hearts
- less cancer
- less diabetes
- leaner bodies
- smarter brains
- better behavior
- less depression
- longer and healthier lives
- fewer "-itis" diseases (e.g., gingivitis, colitis, dermatitis, arthritis)

OIL YOUR GROWING KIDS

Oils, which are really liquid fats, benefit growing bodies and brains because they are:

AWESOME OILS

Four healthy oils that you can feed your family are:

- fish oil
- flaxseed oil
- olive oil
- nut oils, e.g., walnut, almond

- *Nutrient dense.* Oils pack a lot of nutrition into a small volume of food — a perk for finicky eaters.

- *Calorie dense.* Oils contain a lot of calories — a perk for busy kids who don't eat much.

- *Fill-up foods.* A little bit of oil alongside carbs and protein makes a small snack more satisfying — a perk for overeaters.

- *Natural laxatives.* Oils lubricate the intestinal tract — a perk for children who are prone to constipation.

- *Heart healthy.* The healthiest oils lower bad cholesterol and keep arteries healthy.

- *Skin friendly.* Children who eat healthy fats have healthier, more supple skin.

To get more healthy oils into your kids, try these four Sears family favorites:

1. Fish oil. The best source of fish oil is, obviously, fish. But if your children are not fond of seafood, you can use dietary supplements to give them the health benefits of omega 3's. We recommend Neuromins, capsules that supply 200 milligrams of DHA — the healthiest of the omega 3's, especially for growing brains. The DHA in Neuromins is derived from algae (a sea plant), the food the fish eat, so the capsules don't smell or taste fishy. Most young children cannot swallow capsules, so just stick a pin in the capsule and squirt the oil into a smoothie or other snack. (Look for other DHA-enriched foods, too, such as eggs and some cereals.) Valuable information resources for DHA are www.dhadepot.com and www.dhadoc.com.

Fish oil capsules are another source of omega 3's. Most fish oil capsules come in ½-gram to 1-gram doses. For a general guide to how much to take, see page 264. Some fish oil capsules can cause fishy burps. Try camouflaging the oil from a pricked capsule in a smoothie or sauce. Start with a few drops and gradually increase the amount as you shape your children toward accepting fishy tastes. Flavored fish oil capsules and liquid are available; your child may prefer these.

2. Flaxseed oil and flaxseed meal. Omega-3 fats can also be found in plants. Flaxseeds and flaxseed oil are the best plant sources for these healthy oils. Few families seem to know about flaxseeds. Flaxseeds boost immunity; promote cardiovascular, colon, and brain health; and stabilize blood sugar. Flaxseed oil is an excellent natural laxative for kids, far healthier than mineral oil, which is often recommended for constipation but contains no nutrition whatsoever. (It is actually a petroleum product!) Flaxseed meal is made of ground flaxseeds. It gives you all the benefits of the oil plus fiber, and a small amount of protein, vitamins, minerals, and phytonutrients, which have anticancer and immune-boosting properties.

Because flaxseed oil turns rancid easily, buy it in small

amounts and always from the refrigerated section (check the expiration date) and store the container in the refrigerator. Flaxseed meal can be used in baking. Add 1 or 2 tablespoons to muffins or quick breads. But don't use flaxseed oil for cooking, since high heat destroys the health benefits of the oil.

FLAXSEED OIL VS. FISH OIL

Can you expect to get as many health benefits from flaxseed oil as from fish oil? Not exactly. While both are omega-3 fats, the body must take flaxseed oil through a series of biochemical steps before the flaxseed oil becomes DHA that can be utilized by the body. People seem to vary widely in their ability to make this conversion. The DHA in fish oil, on the contrary, is "performed," meaning it needs no biochemical conversion. Because fish oil DHA is a ready-to-use omega-3 fat, its health benefits are nutritionally superior to those of flaxseed oil.

---

3. Olive oil. Unlike fish and flaxseed oil, olive oil doesn't contain significant amounts of omega-3 oil. Its claim to heart-healthy fame is its monounsaturated fats, which decrease levels of bad cholesterol in the blood. As an extra perk, olive oil also contains significant amounts of antioxidants, which strengthen the immune system and help the body repair itself. Because olive oil is made from the flesh of olives rather than from the seeds, it can be processed at lower temperatures, which preserves the nutritional quality of the oil. Here are some helpful tips for adding olive oil to your family's cuisine:

- Buy only virgin or extra virgin olive oil. This designation guarantees that the oil has been processed without heat and chemicals.

Extra virgin is a higher-quality oil — more flavorful and richer in antioxidants.

- For a healthy alternative to butter, use olive oil (with or without a splash of balsamic vinegar) for dipping bread or vegetables.

- Instead of store-bought salad dressings, which are full of sweeteners and chemicals, make your own by adding vinegar and herbs to good-quality olive oil. Whirl it around in the food processor to emulsify the oil so that the dressing will seem more like the commercial products your family may be used to.

- Avoid heating olive oil to high temperatures, such as in deep-fat frying. This can destroy its flavor. Pan-frying or sautéing at moderate heat is a better use for olive oil. If you are using olive oil in a stir-fry, add some water (initially) to keep the oil from getting too hot. Be careful of spattering.

- Olive oil is good for you, but overdosing on it, as with any kind of fats, even healthy ones, can lead to excess body fat. One tablespoon a day is an appropriate amount of olive oil for a school-age child.

4. Nut oils. Oils from almonds, walnuts, hazelnuts, and macadamia nuts are rich sources of heart-healthy, monounsaturated fats. Because studies show that people who eat more almonds have healthier cardiovascular systems, almonds are known as the heart nut. Walnut oil contains some omega-3 fats, so it is known as the brain nut. (Out of its shell a whole walnut actually looks like a tiny brain.) Use these nut oils in salad dressings and dipping sauces. Peanut oil is often used as a cooking oil because it endures heat better than olive oil or vegetable oils. And, of course, older children and adults can also enjoy the benefits of nut oils by eating nuts.

GO RIGHT TO THE SOURCE – SEEDS AND NUTS

If you want to be sure you're getting the most health benefits from oils, eat the nuts and seeds they are extracted from. All kinds of mischief can befall a food as it travels from the farm to processing and finally to the shelf at your supermarket. Bypass the middlemen and you will know more about what your family is eating. You won't have to make sure that the oil wasn't extracted from the plant with heat, which can damage the healthy fats, or chemicals, which you would be better to avoid.

Seeds are packed with fiber and protein, plus vitamins, minerals, and phytonutrients, along with healthy fats. Nut oil may be a concentrated source of fatty acids, but it's not a favorite snack. A handful of almonds, on the other hand, offers a variety of nutrients, with flavor and a satisfying crunch.

Each morning we use our coffee grinder to turn whole flaxseeds into *fresh* flaxseed meal that we mix into our breakfast smoothies or sprinkle on cereal. (See Dr. Bill's smoothie recipe, page 298.) Flaxseeds are more nutritious than flaxseed oil, and grinding your own meal is less expensive than buying it prepackaged. (You have to grind 2 tablespoons of flaxseeds to get about 1 tablespoon of flaxseed oil. All you need is a $20 coffee grinder and a pound of flaxseeds, about $2 at your local nutrition store.)

TRIM THE FAT FROM FAMILY FOODS

Fats that come from meat and poultry sources don't offer the same health benefits as fats from fish and plants. But meat and dairy products are important sources of protein and other nutrients in most families' diets. You and your children can enjoy these foods without putting your arteries at risk if you take care to minimize the amount of fat in these foods. Here are some tips:

- Serve low-fat or nonfat dairy products, organic if possible. (Use whole milk for most toddlers under two.)

- Buy lean meat. Trim away visible fat before cooking.

- Try wild game (e.g., venison, elk, bison), which tends to be higher in healthy fats and lower in fat overall.

- Remove the skin from poultry.

- Serve white meat from poultry. It's leaner than dark; turkey is leaner than chicken.

- Sauté and stir-fry in a small amount of oil rather than frying.

HOW MUCH FAT?

How much fat is enough? How much is too much? Can your diet be too low in fat? As a general guide, healthy children should strive for a diet in which 30 percent of their calories come from fat, 20 percent from protein, and 50 percent from carbohydrates. Saturated fat (fat from animal sources, such as dairy and meat) should make up no more than 7 percent of a child's daily calories. (Unlike with essential fatty acids, found in seafood and plant foods, the body makes saturated fats on its own, so it's not essential that you get them from the foods you eat.) Infants need more concentrated energy than children and adults. Between 40 and 50 percent of the calories in their daily diet should come from fats — which is just the percentage supplied by human milk, the gold standard of infant nutrition.

- Avoid fried foods in restaurants.

- Use olive oil instead of butter for dipping.

- Use full-fat organic yogurt or sour half-and-half in place of sour cream.

NINE WAYS TO CONTROL YOUR CHILD'S CHOLESTEROL

If your family tree is full of people who died of cardiovascular disease, you and your kids are at risk as well. One way you can cut back on the risk is by keeping blood cholesterol levels low. High levels of cholesterol in the blood are associated with an increased risk of heart disease, because cholesterol can damage arteries, causing blockages that become heart disease. Here's a scary statistic: One out of every two children is likely to later develop cardiovascular disease.

Even young children can be affected by high cholesterol levels. Consider these disturbing fat stats: Autopsy studies on accident victims have found fatty streaks in the arteries of children as young as one year of age. These fatty streaks are the beginning of coronary artery disease. Other autopsy studies have shown fat buildup in the coronary arteries of more than half of children between the ages of ten and fourteen.

Clearly, prevention of heart disease should begin in childhood. Children with high cholesterol levels are, of course, more likely to have high cholesterol when they become adults. Here are some cholesterol-lowering tips to keep the heart doctor away:

1. Breastfeed for as long as possible. Studies show that breastfed babies have a lower incidence of heart disease and lower blood cholesterol levels as adults. This is not because they start life on a low-cholesterol diet. They don't. Human milk, like other foods that come from animals, contains significant amounts of cholesterol, while infant formula is cholesterol-free. It may be that the cholesterol in human milk somehow teaches the baby's liver to metabolize cholesterol in a better way. A formula-fed infant misses out on the metabolic programming triggered by the cholesterol in human milk, and so is less able to handle dietary cholesterol later in life.

2. Serve your family more seafood and plant food. Some of the fats in seafood (omega 3's) and plant foods (monosaturated fats) can actually lower cholesterol. Plus, if you're eating more fish, more grains, and more fruits and vegetables, there's less room on your plate for meat, butter, and cheese — the animal-based foods that are high in cholesterol.

3. Cut the cholesterol in foods. When you do serve high-cholesterol foods, trim the fat. Serve lean beef, skinless poultry, and low-fat dairy products.

4. Choose cholesterol-lowering foods. Some plant foods contain sterols, which can reduce the cholesterol absorption from animal foods. These include soy foods (e.g., tofu, soy drinks), high-fiber foods (see page 162), and nuts (especially walnuts).

5. Raise a lean family. As you will learn in chapter 9, being lean means having just the right amount of body fat for your individual body type. Excess body fat can lower the levels of the heart-friendly high-density lipoprotein (HDL), or good cholesterol, and increase the levels of LDL, the artery-clogging low-density lipoprotein, or bad cholesterol. (To remember which cholesterol is good and which is bad, think of LDL as *lousy* cholesterol, and you want it *low;* and HDL as *healthy* cholesterol, and you want it *high.*) Help your kids maintain an appropriate weight and you will also be helping them control their cholesterol.

LIMIT "LIGHT" FOODS

"Light" on a label means the food contains at least one-third fewer calories than the regular version of that same food. This may or may not be a good thing. A "light" version of a high-fat food such as mayonnaise will still contain a lot of fat. And often, when manufacturers lighten up on the amount of fat in a product, they add extra sweeteners and fillers to make up for the flavor and texture that was lost with the reduction in fat. The added sugar ups the carbs and replaces some of the calories eliminated by lowering the amount of fat. Light yogurts are a classical example of this marketing trick. They may contain little or no fat, but they're full of chemical sweeteners.

---

6. Raise young grazers. People who eat frequently, but in small amounts, tend to have lower cholesterol levels. See chapter 6 for information on how to raise a grazer.

7. Raise active kids. You can exercise excess cholesterol right out of your bloodstream! Exercise can increase the good cholesterol and decrease the bad cholesterol and the total cholesterol levels in your blood. Pharmaceutical companies are marketing an increasing number of drugs for lowering cholesterol, but exercise is still the safest way to lower cholesterol, especially in children.

8. Test it. If your child has a family history of early coronary artery disease, or if one or both parents have high cholesterol levels, it's wise to have your doctor check your child's cholesterol levels beginning around five years of age. If the levels are high, changes in diet and exercise can help to bring them down.

9. It starts with YOU. Your kids' arteries are probably decades away from clogging up enough to cause a heart attack or stroke, so there's plenty of time for your healthy changes to take effect. But what about you? Have you had *your* cholesterol checked lately? All it takes is one little finger-prick test at your doctor's office. If going to the doctor scares you, ask your kids' pediatrician to test you the next time you're there with the kids. Dr. Bob was very surprised when he had his cholesterol checked several years ago for a life insurance exam:

> *I was shocked to find out it was 260! I checked it again at my office, and it was even worse — 280! Was I a heart attack waiting to happen? In general, total cholesterol should be below 180. I decided that if I was going to be an active, healthy, energetic grandpa someday and play football with my grandchildren, I would have to make some serious changes now. I started reading labels and stopped eating foods with more than 5 grams of fat per serving (which pretty much cut out all beef, cheese, pastries, ice cream, butter, and anything one would typically eat at a party). I ate fish, lean chicken, and low-fat or nonfat everything (e.g., milk), and snacked on fresh veggies and fruit. For breakfast I ate Whole Oat O's, a cereal with extra oat bran sprinkled on top, along with a smoothie, and drank psyllium husk in water every day. In just a few weeks my cholesterol was down to 177! Since then I've kept it down around 180. I don't have to be as strict with what I eat as I did at the start, but I still have to be sensible.*

Not only do these nine lifestyle and diet changes lower cholesterol, they also lower the other artery-clogging fats, triglycerides, and generally contribute to cardiovascular health. Healthy fats are great grow foods. In the next chapter, you will learn about how to feed your kids more grow foods.

5

Feed Your Kids Grow Foods

When our children were young, we coined the term "grow foods" to explain to them which foods were good to eat and why. Over the years, we've used this phrase in our practice and have found that kids like the term because "grow" is an action word that they associate with getting taller, running faster, becoming smarter, and getting bigger. During nutritional counseling, we have used this term for the past ten years, and it works. Kids want to grow, to get taller and smarter and better at everything, so they react enthusiastically when you explain that certain foods will help them do this. They quickly understand and agree that grow foods or "grow big foods" are good for them.

WHAT'S A GROW FOOD?

Here's what it takes to be a grow food.

It must be nutrient dense. Grow foods have lots of nutrients in every bite relative to the number of calories in the food. For example, ½ cup of raw broccoli provides vitamin A and C, plus fiber, and relatively few calories. A serving of potato chips offers little nutrition but many calories. The broccoli is nutrient dense, and it will help kids grow lean and healthy. The potato chips can, over time, make them fat and sick.

It must be a fill-up food. Grow foods are satisfying and don't leave you feeling sluggish and overly full. Fruits and vegetables are filling, as are high-protein foods. Sweets often leave you wanting more. High-fat foods can make you feel too full. For a list of fill-up foods, see page 156.

It must balance blood sugar levels. Grow foods are digested slowly, so the energy from the food is released into the blood at a steady pace.

It must be free of unhealthy ingredients and artificial additives. These things don't help you grow!

Grow foods are what adults would call whole foods — foods that come from nature, not from factories. Less processing means more nutrients stay in the food. Chemicals that do nothing good and may even be harmful are left out. Everything about a grow food is good for you. Just think of these "nourishing nine" grow foods as those that are eaten in a form close to nature's original:

THE NOURISHING NINE

- eggs
- fruits
- nuts, nut butters
- lean meats, e.g., turkey
- seafood
- tofu
- vegetables, steamed or raw, and legumes, e.g., black beans, peas, lentils
- whole grains
- yogurt, organic

Grow foods pack lots of nutrients into a small volume of food, so kids don't have to eat a lot to get the nutrition they need. This is good news for snackers and kids with small appetites — those kids who don't seem to eat much even though they may eat often. Grow foods are also good for enthusiastic eaters because they tend to be filling and satisfying. It is nearly impossible to overeat when you are eating grow foods, because these foods take up more room in the stomach and are digested slowly. Grow foods help children get on and stay on the right track. Kids learn to associate grow foods with feeling better about themselves and with growing smarter, faster, and healthier. That's the theme of this book. Remember the gut feelings you learned about in chapter 2? Except for children who may be allergic to foods like nuts and dairy, grow foods give good gut feelings. When you start your children on a steady diet of grow foods early in life, there is a good chance that your children will stay on track for the rest of their lives.

Dr. Bob describes what happened when his third child, Joshua, was whining about what was for dinner one night.

> *He began asking for leftovers, remembering that he liked last night's dinner better. "I want leftover broccoli!" he begged. We were happy to comply with his request.*
>
> ◆
>
> *We capitalize on our son's interest in wild creatures by telling him that healthy food will make him a strong creature. He loves the analogy and eats his food right up like a "fierce animal."*

TEACH TRAFFIC-LIGHT EATING

You saw in the last chapter that fats can be categorized by reference to the different-colored signals on a traffic light. In fact, that's true for all foods.

To help your children learn to recognize green-, red-, and yellow-light foods, make a copy of the following chart and hang it on your refrigerator. A more colorful version of the chart is available online at AskDrSears.com/trafficlighteating.

My four-year-old is always asking, "Is this a green-light food or a red-light food?"

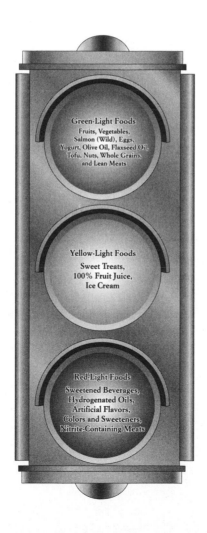

Green-Light Foods
Fruits, Vegetables,
Salmon (Wild), Eggs,
Yogurt, Olive Oil, Flaxseed Oil,
Tofu, Nuts, Whole Grains,
and Lean Meats

Yellow-Light Foods
Sweet Treats,
100% Fruit Juice,
Ice Cream

Red-Light Foods
Sweetened Beverages,
Hydrogenated Oils,
Artificial Flavors,
Colors and Sweeteners,
Nitrite-Containing Meats

TRAFFIC-LIGHT EATING

Green-Light Foods	Yellow-Light Foods	Red-Light Foods
Good for you, enjoy! Eat these grow foods *anytime*.	Slow down, not too much! It's okay to eat these foods *sometimes* as an occasional treat.	Stop and think about a healthier choice! *Never* eat these foods. They are not grow foods.
Beans, cooked, e.g., kidney, lentils, chickpeas	Butter	Beverages sweetened with sugar or corn syrup
Cinnamon	Cakes and cookies, homemade with healthy fats and whole-grain flour	Candy bars, hard candy
Eggs, especially those that have been DHA-enriched	Chocolate, dark	Cold cuts and hot dogs, with nitrites
Fish, especially wild salmon	Frozen yogurt	Fast foods (e.g., french fries, fatty meats)
Flaxseed meal/ flaxseed oil	Fruit juice made from 100 percent juice (without added sweeteners)	Foods with artificial sweeteners
Fruits, all	Honey (not for children under one year)	Foods with dyes and numbers (e.g., red #40) in their ingredients list
Meat, lean		

Green-Light Foods	Yellow-Light Foods	Red-Light Foods
Milk, low-fat, organic	Hot dogs and cold cuts, nitrite free	Foods with hydrogenated oils or shortening
Nut butters, e.g., peanut butter, almond butter	Ice cream	Gelatin desserts with artificial flavors and colors
Nuts (raw)	Maple syrup, pure	
Nut oils	Pasta, white flour	Marshmallows
Olive oil	Pastries and pies made with healthy fats and whole-grain flour	Packaged high-fat, low-fiber bakery goods
Poultry (skinless)	Puddings	Snack foods made with cottonseed oil
Rice, wild or brown	Sour cream	Sodas
Seeds	Whipped cream	
Soybeans	Yogurt, commercially sweetened	
Tofu	White bread	
Turmeric		
Veggies, all		
Wheat germ		
100 percent whole-grain breads and cereals		
Yogurt, low-fat plain or fruit-only		

After teaching kids about traffic-light eating, we frequently notice they start monitoring the eating habits of their parents and grandparents:

When our three-year-old saw my mom eating a hot dog, he commented, "Mama, Grandma eating hot dog. Hot dog red-light food. Not good for you!"

Try not to label food "good" or "bad." This may create guilt or shame around wanting unhealthy foods and set your child up for eating disorders later on. Instead, call foods like broccoli and whole grains "everyday" foods and cookies and cakes "sometimes" foods.

SUPERFOODS FOR KIDS: THE TOP TWELVE

As you can see from the traffic-light chart, veggies, fruits, whole grains, most seafood, lean meats, and low-fat dairy products are grow foods. But some grow foods are packed with more nutritional power than others. Here are our top twelve picks — superfoods that you and your family will enjoy.

Salmon

Salmon is our top superfood pick because it contains many nutrients children need but may not be getting from other foods: omega-3 fats, vitamin B-12, vitamin D, and many other vitamins and minerals. Canned salmon, because it includes the bones (which are soft and okay to eat), is also a rich source of calcium. As we've discussed elsewhere, scientific studies show that the omega-3 fats in salmon (and other fatty fish) improve the functioning of just about every organ in the body. Eating more fish, es-

GO WILD!

You pick up a piece of wild salmon at the market. You notice it's one or two dollars a pound more than the farmed salmon on the next row. Is it worth the extra price? Answer: What's your child's heart health worth? Try this experiment: Compare fillets of wild and farmed salmon. Notice the wild salmon is deeper pink and firm. The farmed fish is pale and flabby. Here are the main reasons to feed your family wild fish:

- *Wild fish is safer.* (See Safe Seafood, page 102.)

- *Wild fish is healthier* for two main reasons. First, wild salmon has a healthier fatty-acid profile. It is higher in the heart- and brain-healthy omega-3 fats DHA and EPA, and lower in the fatty acid AA, which in excess can promote inflammation. In farmed salmon the reverse is true: higher in AA, and lower in DHA and EPA. Second, the rich pink color of wild salmon is due to the powerful antioxidant astazanthin (see all about antioxidants, page 272). The pinkish color of farmed salmon comes from a food coloring that has been added to the fish food. But farmed salmon is still way better than no salmon!

  Use common sense. Which fish should you put into your body — the salmon that swam thousands of miles and ate healthy food, or the fish that paddled around in a pond and ate junk food all day?

pecially salmon, lowers your children's risk of just about every disease, including diabetes, stroke, heart attack, cancer, and high blood pressure.

Serve your family salmon (or other healthy fish; see page 98) at least once a week. For the best flavor and the most nutrition, don't overcook it. Bake, broil, poach, or grill, but don't fry it. Salmon burgers are a healthy alternative to beef burgers. (See our salmon recipes on pages 309, 313, and 314.)

Blueberries

Blueberries contain vitamin C, vitamin E, and fiber, yet their main claim to nutritional fame is their high level of antioxidants called flavonoids. Like other antioxidants, flavonoids play an important part in preventing wear and tear on the tissues of the body, especially in the brain. Blueberries deserve to be called "brain berries." Here's a list of what the antioxidants in blueberries (and other foods high in antioxidants) can do for you:

- reduce the risk of cancer
- clear arteries of plaque and reduce clotting, which improves blood flow and cardiovascular health
- reduce tissue inflammation, which can be the beginning of any number of diseases
- improve neurotransmitter function in the brain
- destroy harmful bacteria
- keep the body younger
- improve eyesight
- protect the intestinal lining from disease

Wild blueberries are more flavorful and tend to be richer in antioxidants, but even cultivated blueberries offer lots of health benefits. Here are some delicious ways to eat blueberries:

- Put a handful of blueberries on or in pancakes.
- Add blueberries to smoothies.
- Mix blueberries with cereal or plain yogurt.
- Make blueberry muffins.

- Add blueberries to green salads.
- Combine blueberries with other fruits in a fruit salad.
- Bake a blueberry pie.
- Mix blueberries and plain yogurt into oatmeal.

(See the related section Berry Good Brains, page 183, and our recipes that use blueberries in chapter 12.)

Spinach

Spinach supplies fiber, vitamin C, vitamin E, calcium, and especially folic acid, or folate, which helps maintain proper growth and function of the central nervous system. Folic acid is especially important for women before and during the first three months of pregnancy, when it has an important role in the prevention of birth defects. Spinach is also rich in the antioxidant lutein, which boosts the health of the retina. We call spinach the "eye and brain green."

Dr. Jim noticed that sharing a meal with another "pure family" can be a way to discover new healthy recipes:

On a recent lecture tour I was on, my family and I spent three days with some friends. In the course of the visit, we tried several healthy new foods and recipes. I couldn't help noticing that my kids complained much less about "yucky" foods than they do at home, and that they were more open to trying new foods when other kids were eating them.

NUTSHELL

Greener greens are better grow foods. The greener the greens, the more nutrients in them!

Romaine lettuce, another dark green leafy vegetable, is a close nutritional second

LETTUCE LESSONS

Shape your children's tastes toward liking a variety of salad greens. Iceberg lettuce, the head lettuce that has the main role in so many restaurant salads and salad bars, ranks at the bottom of the list of healthy greens. We call it "see-through lettuce." Its leaves hold very little nutritional value. Besides, if you eat only iceberg lettuce, you miss out on other tasty, tender greens. Here are some greens that will add variety and flavor to your salads, ranked from most nutritious to least:

- spinach
- arugula
- bok choy
- watercress

- romaine / leaf lettuce
- Boston lettuce, Bibb lettuce
- iceberg

to spinach. It contains as much folate as spinach. Swiss chard, kale, and bok choy are other nutritious greens that can be eaten in salads or cooked. All of these are much more nutritious than wimpy iceberg lettuce.

Nuts

Go nuts! Nuts make our superfood list because they are high in healthy fats, vitamin E, protein, fiber, calcium, iron, and many other vitamins and minerals. In fact, nuts are one of the most nutrient-dense foods you can find. They are the perfect snack food — just a palmful of nuts will satisfy your hunger. Almonds, pecans, pistachios, and walnuts are especially high in vitamin E, a nutrient that many kids lack in their diet. Nuts are not a low-fat food, but the fat in them is the right kind of fat. Seeds have a nutritional value similar to nuts. Sunflower seeds are a favorite addition to salads or trail mix. As a perk, seeds and nuts often make kids thirsty, so they drink more water.

It's hard to recommend one nut over another or give a "Top Nut" award, because each variety represents a uniquely valuable combination of nutrients. Walnuts are highest in omega-3 fats, almonds in vitamin E, and peanuts (which are really legumes, not nuts) in protein and folate. Try these nut-serving tips:

Raw is best. Roasted nuts tend to be the most flavorful but are less nutritious. Buy dry-roasted unsalted nuts that don't have added fat. As a compromise, try half raw and half roasted.

Combine them. In order to take advantage of the unique nutrients in each variety of nut, combine them. Make your own mixed nuts from almonds, walnuts, hazelnuts, cashews, pistachios, chestnuts, and pecans. (See the trail mix recipe on page 302.)

Enjoy nuts ground into nut butter. There are many kinds of nut butter beyond everyday peanut butter. Try almond butter or cashew butter on your toast in the morning. Tahini, which is made from ground sesame seeds, is another tasty alternative to peanut butter.

Keep nuts handy. If you put a bowl of nuts (e.g., shelled walnuts) on the kitchen counter, every time your kids walk by, they may grab a few. Even if they are not fond of nuts, they may eat them simply because they're there!

Prevent choking. Nuts and seeds present a choking hazard for young children, so reserve them for children over three years of age. Infants and toddlers can enjoy nut butters, spread thinly on bread or mixed into other foods. Globs of nut butters can be chokable.

Watch for allergies. If there is a family history of peanut allergy, wait until your child is two years of age before introducing him to peanut butter. (Allergic reactions to nuts are more common and severe in children under two.)

My son loves ground almond "Play-Doh."

WHAT'S IN *YOUR* PEANUT BUTTER?

If you are buying smooth and creamy peanut butter at a regular grocery store, it's probably filled with hydrogenated fats and sugar. Natural, healthy peanut butter has only one ingredient — peanuts. It has no sugar and no hydrogenated oils. It's just pure protein and healthy fats. Natural peanut butter (without added hydrogenated oils) has a thin layer of oil on top, which requires mixing into the rest. If you don't see this separated oil, beware.

Start your kids on healthy peanut butter when they're young and they'll never know the difference. If your kids are older and already hooked on the junk, you may have a hard time winning them over. Smart manufacturers now make a healthier smooth and creamy peanut butter. It still has sugar, but it contains no hydrogenated oils. This may be a good compromise.

Eggs

Eggs are a power-packed food. With a mere 75 calories, they contain 6 grams of protein, plus a small amount of vitamins and minerals. The combination of fat and protein in an egg gives it a high satiety factor, too, so your child feels satisfied when eggs are part of a meal or snack. Egg whites are among the highest-quality proteins. Try these egg tips:

Buy DHA-enriched eggs. DHA is one of the omega-3 fatty acids that are so good for your brain and body. Hens that are fed diets rich in the omega-3 fat DHA lay what are now called "omega eggs" — eggs with greater amounts of DHA.

Whenever possible, buy free-range, organic chicken eggs. Eggs, like chicken meat, reflect the quality of the food the hen eats.

Limit the number of eggs if you have high cholesterol. Even though eggs are high in cholesterol, studies have shown that eating eggs does not contribute to higher blood cholesterol levels in most individuals. But adults and children who already have high cholesterol should limit the number of eggs they eat.

Cook eggs thoroughly. To avoid salmonella infections, be sure to cook eggs thoroughly.

Prepare eggs in a variety of ways. There are many ways to enjoy eggs besides scrambled or sunny side up. Add slices of hardboiled eggs to salads to boost the protein content. Cook eggs with vegetables to make a savory frittata for lunch or dinner.

Tofu

Tofu is made from soy milk, just as cheese is made from cow's milk. In some families, tofu has become the new "cheese." Tofu is terrific because it supplies protein, calcium, zinc, iron, folic acid, and also a bit of B vitamins. The blend of protein, carbs, and healthy fats (and even some fiber) in tofu makes it a food that gives you a good, satisfied gut feeling, not the kind of food that leaves you feeling bloated or sluggish. In fact, soy foods, especially tofu and soy "nuts," are all-purpose health foods. Soy builds healthy hearts and bones and reduces cancer risk, mainly

SNEAKY TIPS TO GET NUTRIENTS INTO YOUR FAMILY'S FOOD

- Sprinkle a little cinnamon on everything you can (e.g., yogurt, applesauce, cereal, oatmeal cookies, pudding, and baked goods). For the health benefits of cinnamon, see page 84.

- Replace white flour with whole wheat pastry flour in your family's favorite recipes. Whole wheat pastry flour has a finer texture than regular whole wheat flour, so it is more consistent with that of white flour. Or go half and half on the flours (or even three-quarters white to one-quarter whole wheat) until your family gets used to the whole wheat flavor and texture. They may not even notice, if you don't tell.

- Dice raw leafy greens very, very small and sprinkle them into spaghetti sauce. Try to use ones that they won't usually eat, like kale or spinach. You can even chop them in a food processor. Just 1 tablespoonful per day can make a difference over time.

- Blend some organic spinach or chard into a fruit-and-yogurt smoothie.

- Add omega-3 oils to foods by using them in salad dressings, tossing pasta with them, or mixing them into individually served soups, chili, or other foods that are good hiding places. (Don't overheat the oil.)

- Use whole-grain pasta noodles, such as whole wheat or brown rice pasta. Soy pasta can also be mixed in to add protein. Soy pasta tends to have a very different texture than the others; mixing it with another pasta can mask it.

- To get more protein into a picky eater, add protein powder to hot or cold cereal, smoothies, juice, or baked goods. Even a gram here and there adds up.

- For children under four, grind chokable foods, such as nuts and seeds (flax and sunflower), in a coffee grinder and add them to oatmeal, smoothies, or salads.

- Use fruits, juice, a little honey, or Xylitol as a sweetener. Concentrated fruit juices such as apple or white grape also work well as a replacement for sugar or corn syrup in many recipes. Or at least use half sugar and half juice concentrate to cut down on refined sugar.

- Add diced vegetables to kid favorites such as mac and cheese. Scatter them on top of pizza or add them to soup.

- Use a variety of healthy dips to entice raw vegetable eating: hummus, guacamole, yogurt dip, peanut butter, bean dip, salsa, and olive oil.

- Dilute fruit juice with water to cut down on the surge of sugar. Add a splash of vegetable juice into the fruit juice. Carrot juice is great in apple juice. For younger children who still use sippy cups, try using colored cups to mask the color of the juice. They won't know if their juice is a little green from a splash of spinach juice mixed in.

because of the phytoestrogens in soy. (The health benefits of phytos are explained in chapter 8, Feed Your Family Immune-Boosting Foods.) Population studies have found an association between longevity and diets high in soy foods. Soy foods enjoy a low glycemic index and contain nutrients called fructooligosaccharides (FOS), which nourish beneficial intestinal bacteria.

Tofu tips. You can buy soft tofu or firm tofu, which contain varying degrees of moisture. (Firm tofu has less.) Tofu is a versatile food. You can blend soft tofu into smoothies, add chunks of firm tofu to a stir-fry, purée it into dips and spreads, and even serve it in cubes as a finger food for toddlers or an ingredient in salads and soup. Tofu tends to take on the taste of the foods it's mixed with, so it's easy to sneak it into your family's diet. We put tofu in our family smoothies each morning, and the kids can't even tell it's there.

Yogurt

Yogurt is a favorite of many kids and adults. It's high in protein and calcium, and it's easier to digest than milk, which is important for family members who may be lactose intolerant. The live bacterial cultures in yogurt help keep intestines healthy, and yogurt also offers a boost to the immune system.

Yogurt is a convenient and versatile grow food. You can eat it straight from the container or combine it with many other foods. Here are some ideas:

- Add yogurt to fruit smoothies.
- Put a dollop on warm oatmeal or eat it with cold cereal in place of milk.
- Mix yogurt with fruit and put it in the freezer. Take it out when it's only partially frozen and stir, and you have a gelato-like frozen dessert.

- Use full-fat yogurt instead of sour cream on baked potatoes, burritos, and fajitas.
- Mix yogurt with herbs and spices to make dips and salad dressings.

Yogurt-buying tips. Buy plain low-fat or nonfat yogurt, organic if possible, and add your own fruit and flavorings. Most of the fruit-flavored yogurt on the shelf at the supermarket contain enough sugars, sweeteners, and stabilizers to partially negate the nutritional value of the yogurt. Usually the shorter the list of ingredients, the healthier the yogurt. The healthiest yogurt contains only milk and "bugs" — the active bacterial cultures that turn milk into yogurt. Look for the phrase *live, active cultures,* which means that a certain amount of live, active bacterial cultures were put in the yogurt at the time of manufacturing but after pasteurization. Remember, the 13 to 15 grams of "sugars" listed on the label of plain yogurt are lactose and count as good carbs.

Avocados

Avocados are another nutrient-dense food on our list of top grow foods. Avocados, like olives, are one of the few foods that are both rich in healthy fats and free of cholesterol. The fats in the avocado are primarily the heart-healthy monounsaturated type, and this nutrient-rich fruit even contains a bit of the healthiest fat, omega 3. Eating these healthy fats reduces the level of unhealthy fats in the bloodstream. Avocados also contain significant amounts of B vitamins, vitamin E, and folate, as well as fiber. Try these buying and serving tips:

Buy avocados that are not yet ripe. They should be firm but not hard. When you press the avocado, your fingers should not leave a dent.

Ripen avocados at home. When you get home from the market, place avocados in a paper bag and store them at room temperature until they are soft enough to eat, but not too soft. Then keep them refrigerated to slow the ripening if you need them to keep until later.

Serve avocados as a snack. Run a knife lengthwise around the avocado, from top to bottom and bottom to top, cutting all the way through to the pit. Then hold the avocado in both hands and twist at the cut. The halves should separate easily, leaving the pit in one half. Let your child spoon out the flesh from the seedless half. To use the rest later, sprinkle the cut surface of the seeded half with lemon juice and store it in a plastic bag. Use within a day or two. Placing the pit in the bowl of guacamole will help it stay fresh.

Mash it up. Mashed avocado makes great baby food. Introduce it as one of your infant's first foods. It has a smooth texture and lots of nutrients in every spoonful.

Use it in a dip or as a spread for toddlers and young children, or spice it up and make guacamole for older kids and adults.

Oatmeal

Oatmeal continues to be a favorite family food of both little and big people. It's high in protein and provides many vitamins and minerals. The heart-healthy fiber found in oatmeal helps lower cholesterol and stabilize blood sugar. Here are some buying and serving suggestions:

Serve steel-cut oats. These 100 percent whole-grain oats are cut, not rolled. They have a hearty texture and are the most flavorful oatmeal.

Avoid instant oatmeal. The extra processing of the grain removes some of the nutrients, and it's loaded with sugar. (See related discussion of instant foods on page 193.)

Cook oatmeal in a Crock-Pot. To treat your busy, modern family to an old-fashioned, slow-cooked oatmeal breakfast, use a Crock-Pot. You can cook the oatmeal during the night and treat your family to hot oatmeal in the morning. For a delicious combination, add a couple of tablespoons of frozen blueberries that have been thawed, a sprinkling of cinnamon, and a dollop of plain yogurt (instead of butter). The yogurt seems to "melt," adding a creamy texture.

Flaxseeds

Flaxseeds belong on every family's grow-foods list. Flaxseeds contain protein, healthy fat, fiber, B vitamins, folate, and minerals. They are also rich in phytos that help the immune and cardiovascular systems and fight cancer.

Flaxseeds are too small to chew, so put 1 or 2 tablespoons in a coffee grinder and grind for five or ten seconds to make flaxseed meal, which you can then sprinkle on cereal, put in a smoothie, add to a salad, or mix into muffin batter. Be aware that when mixed into a liquid, flaxseed meal thickens or congeals somewhat. One tablespoon of flaxseed meal a day is a healthy amount for a young child, 2 tablespoons for an older child or adult.

Beans

Beans such as kidney beans and black beans are a kid-friendly food that can be added to salads, puréed into dips, and added to soups and chili. Beans contain more protein and fiber than any other vegetable, so they are a great fill-up food, helping children

WHY WHOLE GRAINS?

Whole grains are a whole lot more nutritious than processed grains, especially wheat. A kernel of wheat has three parts: The outer layer, the wheat bran, is highest in fiber and valuable minerals and vitamins. At the heart of the kernel is the wheat germ, which is not very big but still contains a lot of the protein, along with minerals and vitamins, especially vitamin E. The third and largest part of the wheat kernel is called the endosperm. It contains most of the carbohydrates and protein but not much else. White flour, also known as wheat flour, is made only from the endosperm. *Whole* wheat flour includes the bran and the germ — it is made from the whole wheat kernel. It is a good source of fiber, vitamins, and minerals, as well as carbs and protein. Because the bran and germ were removed from the wheat kernel before it was ground into flour, white flour has to be enriched. The manufacturers add vitamins and minerals to make up for what was lost, but they don't add back as much of some nutrients as they take out. For example, even after the white bread is "enriched," it has less vitamin E, vitamin B-6, magnesium, fiber, zinc, and potassium than whole wheat bread. The white bread also has 75 percent less fiber, giving it a higher glycemic index than the whole wheat bread. The carbs in the white bread will be absorbed into the bloodstream more quickly, where they can make trouble. (See Healthy Carbs vs. Junky Carbs, page 75, and more about "air bread" on page 246.)

feel satisfied without eating too much. Other foods in the legume family, such as peas, lentils, and chickpeas, contain even more protein, fiber, folate, B vitamins, and minerals than kidney and black beans, yet many kids prefer plain old beans. Incorporate beans and other legumes into your family menus, so that your kids learn to like and appreciate them.

You have to read the label carefully to find out if bread and other baked goods are made from whole grains. You can't tell by the color of the bread, since brown bread may simply be white bread colored with molasses. Bread described on the label as whole grain may be 50 percent whole grain, with the other 50 percent being processed white flour. Even the term "multigrain" is ambiguous, since a multigrain product may contain not whole grains but just multiple kinds of processed grains. To be sure you are getting the best nutrition, look for the words "100 percent whole grain" on the label and "whole wheat" in the list of ingredients.

It's hard to get whole grains into kids whose tastes have been shaped toward liking doughy, smooth white bread. Make whole wheat bread and pasta and whole-grain cereals the standard in your family, so that your children's tastes are shaped to enjoy grains that have some substance. They will come to prefer these whole-grain foods and enjoy better health when they are older. (See the related section on shopping for cereals, page 245.)

Besides whole wheat, other whole grains to look for include oatmeal, rye, millet, barley, amaranth, spelt, and quinoa. Brown rice has more fiber than the more highly processed white rice, and wild rice has more fiber than brown rice.

Tomatoes

Tomatoes make it onto our Top Twelve list not only because they are nutritious but also because they are part of so many foods and combinations of food that kids like. When you look at charts

---

SUPER SPRINKLES

Kids love sprinkles (especially the chocolate kind). Capitalize on this fun food idea! To shape your toddler's taste for these foods, grind nuts and seeds in a coffee grinder for about ten seconds (nuts and seeds are chokable foods for children under three or four). Try these healthy sprinkle choices:

- flaxseed meal
- cinnamon for "sweet" (for its health benefits, see page 84)
- turmeric for "savory" (see page 207)
- ground almonds (call it "crunchies")
- ground sunflower seeds
- protein powders with multivitamins and multiminerals, chocolate- or vanilla-flavored
- fresh lemon or lime juice
- lemon peel
- ginger

---

showing amounts of this or that vitamin, other veggies may outshine tomatoes, but try getting kids to eat kale. Tomatoes are a good source of fiber and vitamin C, plus they contain some B vitamins and minerals. What makes tomatoes special is their intense red color, a sign that they are rich in phytonutrients, including lycopene, a top antioxidant. Cooking tomatoes enables more of the lycopene to be absorbed. Try these tomato-serving tips:

- Serve them in sauces, purées, salsas, and juice.

- Serve tomato-based foods (e.g., spaghetti sauce) with a fat, such as olive oil. Fat helps the body absorb antioxidants into the bloodstream.

TOP GROW FOODS BY CATEGORY

Here's a shopping list of nutrient-rich grow foods that kids will eat and love.

Dairy Products
cottage cheese
milk, organic, low-fat
yogurt, plain, low-fat

Fruits
avocados
blueberries
papayas

Grains
amaranth
oats
whole wheat bread
wild rice

Meats/Poultry
top-round steak, lean
turkey
wild game

Nuts
almonds
peanuts
walnuts

Oils
flaxseed oil
nut oils
olive oil

Seafood
cod
halibut
trout
tuna
salmon, wild

Seeds
pumpkin
sesame
sunflower

Soy Foods
edamame
(fresh, cooked soybeans)
soy beverages
tofu

Vegetables
beans, e.g., lentils, chickpeas
spinach
tomatoes

You can mix many of these grow foods together in a grow-food salad (see recipe, page 308).

PACK ON THE PROTEIN

Protein is an important grow food. Growing bodies need protein in order to build, repair, and maintain body tissues. Consider these protein perks:

Protein perks up the brain. Neurotransmitters, highly specialized chemicals that carry messages in the brain and throughout the body, are made up of protein. It's important to have the right protein on hand to construct these important chemicals. The better you feed the brain, the better it can do everything from math problems to controlling impulsive behavior. A high-protein breakfast will help both students and parents perform well all morning long.

Protein is a feel-good food. Protein leaves the gut feeling satisfied. There's a chemical explanation for this: Protein is the prime ingredient of dopamine, a feel-good neurotransmitter found in the intestines. Dopamine helps you feel satisfied and content after a snack or meal.

Protein is a fill-up food. Protein is filling. Kids may go overboard eating carbs or high-fat foods, but it's hard to overeat protein-rich foods. Like foods high in fiber, protein foods fill you up without overeating. For this reason, high-protein snacks and meals are ideal for people who are trying to lose weight. Protein is a more-for-less food — more nutritious but less fattening. Unlike when you eat carbs, you won't be hungry again an hour after eating foods with a lot of protein.

Try this experiment. Use a blender to make a smoothie with just fruit juice and fruit, which are nearly all carbs. Notice that you have to drink a lot of this to feel satisfied. You'll also find that you get hungry again soon. The next time you have a craving for a fruit smoothie, make it with plain yogurt as well as fruit. Since yogurt is a protein food, you will probably notice this smoothie keeps you satisfied longer. Next, to really boost the protein content of this smoothie, add 1 tablespoon of peanut butter, which contains both protein and healthy fat. This makes a smoothie that's really a meal.

Protein revs up your metabolism. Did you know that your body has to burn calories to digest the food you eat? The body uses more than twice as many calories to digest protein as it does to digest fat and carbs. Another way of saying this is that protein has a high thermic effect, meaning that the body has to use energy just to digest the food. This speeds up your metabolism, helping your body burn more calories.

Protein steadies blood sugar. Protein is digested slowly, so the energy from a meal high in protein enters your bloodstream at a slow, steady rate. Your body responds by releasing insulin steadily. As a result, you don't experience the blood sugar highs and lows that you get from eating junk carbs all by themselves. Protein promotes hormonal harmony in the body and brain, so you and your children can meet life's ups and downs in a calm, steady way. Because of its filling and blood sugar–stabilizing features, protein is an ideal snack food.

Best Protein Foods for Your Family

Unlike some carbs and fats, there is no such thing as an unhealthy protein. Still, some proteins are more nutritious than others. Proteins are made up of substances called amino acids, and the body can use certain kinds of amino acids more efficiently than others. For example, the amino acids found in human milk are exactly the type that human infants need as building blocks to grow healthy skin, strong bodies, and alert little brains. Protein foods that contain more of the really useful amino acids are said to have a high biological value. Here's how proteins rank according to their biological value:

- whey protein (the main protein in human milk and protein extracts from dairy products)
- eggs
- fish
- dairy products
- beef and poultry
- soy
- legumes (e.g., lentils, beans)

Another way to rank protein foods is by their protein density, the percentage of protein in a particular food relative to the total number of calories in that food. Compare the protein density of the foods in the chart on the facing page.

As you can see from the chart, foods that contain more fat or carbs have a lower protein density. But even foods near the bottom of the chart make satisfying meals and snacks — because they contain some protein.

Another way to rank protein foods is by the company they keep. A greasy cheeseburger is not a good choice for lunch, because it's a fat protein. Tuna is a "lean protein"; it has less overall fat, and the fat in tuna is a healthy fat. Cereals can be a good source of protein. They are low in fat, and cereal protein comes packaged with healthy fiber. However, cereals that are full of sugar and contain artificial flavors and colors do not provide the kind of protein food that helps kids grow.

Here's a way to tell your kids which protein is the leanest: *Pro-*

FOODS THAT PACK THE MOST PROTEIN

Food	Grams of Protein per Serving	Percentage of Calories as Protein
Fish, salmon and tuna (4 ounces)	25–30	83
Egg white (1)	3.5	82
Cottage cheese, nonfat (½ cup)	15	75
Poultry, breast, no skin (4 ounces)	25	75
Kidney beans (½ cup)	7	60
Tofu, firm (3 ounces)	13	45
Yogurt, plain nonfat (1 cup)	12	40
Beef, lean (4 ounces)	30	40
Egg, whole (1)	6	33
Milk, 1 percent (8 ounces)	8	32
Peanut butter (2 tbsp.)	8	17
Cereal (1 cup) with ½ cup milk	6–8	17
Nuts or sunflower seeds (1 ounce)	7	16
Pasta, whole-grain (1 cup)	7	15
Whole wheat bread (1 slice)	3	15

tein from fish that swim or from plants that grow in the fields is the healthiest.

How Much Protein Should Your Family Eat?

As a general guide, we advise parents to encourage children aged six to twelve to eat ¾ to 1 gram of protein per pound per day. For example, if your child weighs 50 pounds, strive for an average of 40 to 50 grams of protein a day. A child does not have to eat a lot of food to get this much protein, as you can see from the chart

---

PLAY SHOW AND TELL!

Try this salmon versus sirloin game to explain lean protein and fat protein to your children. Go to your usual supermarket and purchase a piece of sirloin steak. Next, go to a specialty market and buy some wild salmon. Then sit down with your child and compare the two. "Notice the sirloin is flabby (even though it's a high-protein food) and marbled with all that white stuff, which is fat. Fat makes muscles weak. This steak came from an animal that sat around and ate junk food all day. If you eat junk food, you get junk muscle. Now feel and see the difference in the meat that came from the fish who swam upstream and ate healthy food all day. It looks and feels strong. Which do you want your muscles to look like?"

---

above. This means that 20 to 25 percent of a child's daily calories should come from protein. The minimum amount of protein that your child needs is ½ gram per pound per day, according to the USDA's recommended daily values, but we think it's a good idea to strive for more protein in his diet. Otherwise, kids are likely to eat too many carbs and too much fat. Kids need extra protein during the growth spurts of early childhood and adolescence and when they participate in strenuous sports activities. As kids approach adult size, the proportional need for protein lessens. Adults and teens should strive for ½ to ¾ gram of protein per pound of ideal weight per day. Teens who are participating in weight training may need more.

Do the math! Your daily diet is composed of three nutrients: protein, fat, and carbohydrates. The more calories you get from protein, the fewer you need from fat and carbohydrates. Remember our suggested balance: 50 percent carbs, 20 to 25 percent protein, and 25 to 30 percent healthy fats. Protein tends to keep you lean; excess fat and carbs are more easily stored as excess fat. When your body has more protein than it can handle, it simply disassembles the protein, keeps the amino acids it needs, and discards the rest in the urine. The body can't store excess dietary protein as easily as it can store excess fat and carbs.

6

Raise a Grazer

Big meals can cause big biochemical problems. They can also cause indigestion. Overwhelm your intestines with a big meal and you may feel uncomfortable for hours. Pay attention to that bloated, crampy feeling. Your stomach is trying to tell you that it would be a lot happier if you would graze your way through the day. We want to help you and your children get used to the comfortable feeling of grazing rather than always filling up at each meal.

By the word *grazing* we mean eating frequent mini-meals throughout the day. Wise grazers eat good food, in the right balance of carbs, protein, and fat, so that they stay lean. When you graze, you don't wait until you're ravenously hungry to eat. You eat every couple hours, and the steady supply of energy you get from frequent small meals helps to steady your blood sugar levels and keep your insulin levels stable.

GRAZERS VS. GORGERS

Grazers Are . . .	Gorgers Are . . .
• likely to be lean	• likely to be fat
• more satisfied, less hungry	• more hungry, less satisfied
• clearer thinkers	• foggier thinkers
• less moody	• likely to have mood swings
• more alert	• sleepier
• more energetic	• less energetic
• more comfortable in their guts	• frequently suffering from indigestion
• healthier physically	• at greater risk for diabetes and cardiovascular disease

GRAZING IS FILLING WITHOUT BEING FATTENING

At first, it may not seem to make sense that people who eat more often can actually be leaner than those who eat only three meals a day. But studies show that people who graze on good food tend to eat fewer total calories during the day. Consequently, they tend to be leaner. Because grazers are never desperately hungry, they eat less. When you get into a routine of grazing before you get really hungry rather than eating after you get hungry, you tend to be satisfied with less food. If you regularly feed your stomach less food, it starts to feel full with a lower volume of food. You may have heard that you can shrink your stomach by eating less. Animal studies suggest that there is some anatomic truth to this idea. Kids who are used to grazing on mini-meals don't overload themselves with food, even when presented with the opportunity to do so.

Grazing is at the heart of good metabolic programming for

SCIENCE SAYS: GRAZERS TEND TO BE HEALTHIER

Here's a summary of what researchers have learned about the benefits of grazing. Grazers tend to:

- *Have more stable blood sugar and insulin levels.* Grazing promotes insulin efficiency, while overeating contributes to the development of insulin-resistant diabetes.

- *Be leaner.* Studies show that people who eat more frequent smaller meals tend to consume fewer calories than those who eat less frequent larger meals. The body burns fat after smaller meals but stores fat after large ones. Obesity researchers refer to this as adaptive hyperlipogenesis, which simply means the body gets used to processing big meals by storing a larger amount of body fat.

- *Show fewer mood swings.* Stable blood sugars mean fewer food cravings and more stable moods. Levels of cortisol (stress hormones) tend to be lower in grazers than in gorgers.

your child's body. Once your child's body and brain get used to the steady insulin and blood sugar levels that come with grazing, he'll make this eating pattern a way of life. When grazers depart from their usual way of eating and eat too much at one meal — for example, during a vacation or at a special holiday meal — they feel very uncomfortable later. The groggy, overfull sensations remind them that they are happier when they eat less food but more often.

Be aware that overgrazing can make you overfat. For example, having a big bowlful of nuts beside you and mindlessly munching on them while you're reading can lead to excess weight gain.

- *Experience less acid reflux.* Grazers tend to suffer less from heartburn or acid reflux disease. A big meal increases pressure in the stomach, triggering the regurgitation of stomach contents and stomach acids back up into the esophagus. Eating less food at one time can keep this from happening.

- *Have a lower risk of cardiovascular disease and atherosclerosis.* Grazers have lower blood cholesterol. Heart attacks and strokes commonly occur after a big meal, when the heart becomes stressed by having to pump harder and faster. A sudden spike in blood fat levels caused by gorging on a high-fat meal (called after-meal lipemia) can cause arteries to go into spasm, slowing blood flow to vital organs such as the heart and the brain.

- *Have less inflammation throughout their bodies.* Inflammation damages cells and organs, leading to "-itis" illnesses. (See Don't Raise an iBod, page 38.)

However, snacking on a palmful of nuts can promote weight control.

MAKE GRAZING DOABLE

We realize that eating styles are highly personal, and it may be difficult for many families to make the changes we suggest. We want to help you get started. Let's say you are convinced by the studies on the health benefits of grazing, but your lifestyle, your work, and your child's school schedule make everyday grazing impractical for you and your kids. Or you may feel fine on your present three-square-meals eating pattern. You may wonder how you can actually do this grazing thing in your real world and make it work for you and your kids. While we present the ideal, we realize that every family must do what works for them. Here are some ideas for making grazing work:

- Make a shopping list for trail mix, smoothies, and snack foods (see recipes in chapter 12).

- Start with one change such as drinking a smoothie (see The Sipping Solution on page 166) or nibbling on trail mix as your snack. After you get a feel for how this change helps you, and your body is convinced, make even more changes.

- Eat smaller portions at your "three squares."

- Make healthier food choices for both snacks and meals.

- Take a water bottle with you and sip frequently.

WELCOME THE WELLNESS HORMONE – INSULIN

Question: What are the three most important words that describe the feeling of being in biochemical balance? Answer: "stable insulin levels." Grazing keeps body and brain in biochemical balance by keeping insulin levels stable. We call insulin the "wellness hormone" or the "health hormone," because when insulin levels are just right, the whole body feels healthier. When a child's insulin is stable, so is his behavior likely to be. Here's our Insulin 101 Course — information that will help you understand why so much of the eating plan presented in this book is geared toward maintaining steady levels of sugar and insulin in the blood.

Insulin balances blood sugar. Cells need carbs. As your food is digested and absorbed, your blood sugar level rises, which triggers the pancreas to release insulin. Insulin then travels to the cells, where it acts like a key, opening doors on the cell membrane that let the sugar in so that it can be used as fuel.

But what happens when too much glucose hits the bloodstream all at once? The cells respond to this glucose overload by not letting insulin open all the doors. The insulin and the blood glucose respond by saying, "Okay, we'll just go somewhere else and hang around in case you need us later." Insulin then helps the glucose molecules pile up on one another to make a larger molecule called glycogen, which is stored in the liver. Then, when the blood sugar level falls too low, insulin stimulates the hormone glucagon, which withdraws the glucose (stored as glycogen) from the glycogen bank in the liver and sends it back into the bloodstream to provide energy for the body. When insulin and glucagon are in balance, the body maintains a steady, optimal blood sugar level.

This is how the system is supposed to work. But suppose excess glucose and insulin storm the doors of the cells day after day. The cells start to resist the excess insulin, and a condition called insulin-resistance, or Type 2 diabetes, develops. Eventually, the cells don't respond to normal amounts of insulin, so the pancreas churns out more. This chronically high level of insulin in the blood, along with elevated glucose levels, can have disastrous effects on health if left untreated. Eventually, the insulin-producing cells of the pancreas may wear out, and people with Type 2 diabetes may need insulin shots, as well as their oral medication, to control the levels of glucose in the blood.

Besides increasing the risk of developing diabetes, high insulin levels in the early years may lead to many other adult diseases. Here's how too much insulin in the blood contributes to obesity, cardiovascular disease, and other chronic health conditions.

Excess insulin stores fat. Insulin is called the storage hormone, storing glucose and fat for later use. If you eat more carbs than your body can burn or store in the liver, the excess has to go somewhere. You guessed it. Excess sugar makes you fat, especially around the abdomen. This is why big middles and Type 2 diabetes tend to go together. Not only do high insulin levels cause excess fat storage, but they also inhibit the release of stored fat. For this reason, it's hard to lose excess body fat when your insulin levels are elevated much of the time from a diet of junk carbs. Healthy eating will give you just the right level of insulin to store just the right amount of body fat for your body type.

Insulin regulates growth hormone. Insulin levels that stay too high for too long interfere with the work of growth hormone. The result may be muscle weakness and less-than-optimal growth. Kids may grow wider instead of taller and stronger.

Insulin affects the cardiovascular system. High insulin levels can raise blood cholesterol levels. (Insulin that remains too high for too long can also reduce levels of HDL, the good cholesterol.) Cholesterol can form plaque that clogs arteries and reduces blood flow to the heart and brain. Autopsy studies have found fatty deposits in the arteries in children as young as one.

Insulin regulates inflammation. If insulin levels are too high for too long, the body reacts with inflammation, which can lead to a host of "-itis" diseases, such as arthritis, colitis, and dermatitis. Remember, don't be an iBod (see page 38).

Five Ways to Keep Your Insulin Stable

High insulin levels and the insulin inefficiency that follows are the biochemical origins of many kinds of "unwellness." One of the best ways you can give your child the gift of health now and in the future is to program the child's body to maintain stable insulin levels. The way your child eats and lives can keep the blood at just the right insulin level and promote the appropriate release of insulin (not too much and not too little). Here are some ways you and your child can avoid insulting the insulin while promoting hormonal harmony in the body:

1. Eat the right carbs. As we said earlier, healthy eating depends on a right-carb diet, not a low-carb diet. Foods with a low glycemic index (see page 80) stimulate a lesser insulin response than those with a high glycemic index. Whether a food is made of just carbs or carbs packaged with protein, fiber, or fat greatly affects the way insulin is released. Carb-only foods (e.g., sweetened beverages) are rapidly absorbed into the bloodstream, causing blood sugar to rise quickly, triggering a steep rise in insulin as well. All that insulin ensures that the sugar is rapidly cleared from the blood, so blood sugar levels fall again, resulting in hunger, carb cravings, and stressed-out behavior. Protein, fat, and fiber partnered with carbs slow their absorption so that the food does not trigger a sugar/insulin rush.

Fructose, the sugar in fruit, boasts a couple of biochemical quirks that make it insulin friendly. (Note: High-fructose corn syrup, despite its name, does not share these same good quirks.) When fructose enters the bloodstream, it goes directly to the liver and does not trigger the insulin cycle. Also, fructose can enter cells directly, as an energy-rich carb, without needing to be escorted by insulin. As an added perk, fructose has a high thermo-

---

HOW TO KEEP YOUR INSULIN LEVELS STABLE

- Eat carbs that come naturally packaged with protein and fiber.
- Do not eat or drink carb-only foods without accompanying them with some protein, fiber, or fat.

---

genic effect, meaning your body burns a lot of calories just digesting it. So when you have a craving for something sweet, choose a piece of fruit rather than a soda or candy bar.

2. Graze on good carbs. Healthy insulin levels depend on not only what carbs you eat but also how you eat them. Grazing on frequent mini-meals throughout the day is more insulin friendly than gorging on big meals. Grazing is an eat-as-you-burn-energy pattern of eating, which helps stabilize insulin.

3. Eat high-fiber foods. Studies have shown that people who eat more fiber tend to have lower and more stable insulin levels. (For the health benefits of fiber, see page 157.)

4. Eat protein with every meal and snack. Protein curbs overeating and therefore keeps insulin levels stable. Eating foods high in protein stimulates the release of the hormone glucagon, and a rise in glucagon levels causes a fall in insulin levels. Making protein a part of every meal and snack you eat stabilizes your blood sugar and consequently your insulin levels.

5. Move. Exercise slows the release of insulin. When you are moving energetically, your body anticipates your need for energy, so cells become more sensitive to insulin. This enables more sugar to get into the cells so that they can keep going. The first "prescription" we write for patients who are developing insulin resistance or "pre-diabetes" is MOVE!

FEED YOUR FAMILY FILL-UP FOODS

Supersize me! It's a great slogan but a bad idea. Supersize portions have led to a supersize nation. Restaurant portions have grown as America's weight problems have grown.

Serving children large portions of high-calorie foods conditions them to overeat, and studies have shown that obese children tend to need more food to fill them up. Eating more food piles on more pounds and perpetuates an unhealthy satiety cycle. Part of shaping your children's tastes and eating habits is to help them feel more satisfied with appropriate amounts of food. To do this, plan your family's menus around foods that fill them up with fewer calories. We call these "fill-up foods." Fill-up foods help you feel full without getting fat. They work with your body's satiety mechanism — the communication system between your gut and your brain that figures out when you've eaten enough and when it is time to eat again.

Generally speaking, the more fiber, protein, and fat, and the

---

OUT OF SIGHT, OUT OF TUMMY

Remember how your grandmother used to warn, "Your eyes are bigger than your stomach"? Some children like the look of big portions. Studies show that they eat more when they are served more. Studies also show that children are satisfied with less food when they are allowed to serve themselves. Maybe kids' eyes know best!

fewer carbs a food contains, the longer it will satisfy you. Fill-up foods are very helpful when you are trying to eat less and control your weight. Here's what to be aware of:

- Fill-up foods tend to be nutrient dense, meaning they pack a lot of nutrition into relatively few calories. In fact, studies show that when people are allowed to eat all they want of nutrient-dense foods, they consume fewer calories than when they are allowed to eat as much as they want of highly refined and processed foods.

- Healthy carbs (those that are partnered with protein and fiber) are more satisfying than junk carbs. (See Healthy Carbs vs. Junky Carbs, page 75.)

- The least satisfying "foods" are carb-only candies and junk carb drinks that are simply sugar and water. Not only do these things fail to fill you up, but eating or drinking them also triggers the release of hormones that stimulate your appetite and make you want to eat more.

FILL-UP FOODS

Apples	Nuts
Avocados	Oatmeal
Beans	Olive oil
Beef	Oranges
Cereals, high-protein, high-fiber	Popcorn
	Potatoes, boiled
Cheese	Salads
Cherries	Seafood
Eggs	Soybeans
Fish	Vegetables
Grapes	Whole-grain breads
Lentils	Whole-grain pasta

- Solid foods tend to be more satisfying than liquid meals (with the exception of homemade vegetable soups and smoothies such as School-Ade, page 298, which include satisfying amounts of protein, healthy carbs, fat, and fiber).

- Fill-up foods tend to contain a lot of water and fiber. Water and fiber increase the bulk of foods without increasing their calorie content. Apples and oranges are good examples of this.

- High-protein meals are generally more satisfying than an equal amount of calories in carbs.

Fill Up Your Family with Fiber

Fiber is the chewable, structural part of fruits, vegetables, and grains that is neither digested nor absorbed by the body. It is calorie-free but takes up lots of room in your stomach. Here's what fiber can do for you and your family:

Fiber keeps you from overeating. High-fiber foods require lots of chewing. Just having food in your mouth sets off feelings of satiety and dampens hunger a bit. So when something takes a long time to chew and swallow, you're likely to eat less overall. (This is why weight-loss programs remind dieters to chew their food longer and take smaller bites.)

Fiber-rich foods are digested more slowly and stay in the stomach longer, so you feel full with less food and stay full longer. Population studies have shown that people who eat more fiber tend to be leaner and healthier. In fact, it's hard to eat a high-fiber diet that isn't healthy, since fiber is found mainly in fruits, vegetables, and whole grains. In one study, people who ate a high-fiber breakfast cereal ate an average of 150 fewer calories per day than those who ate a low-fiber cereal. Eating 150 fewer calories each day translates into 1½ fewer pounds of fat deposited per month. Fiber even soaks up some of the fat you eat, so you absorb fewer

---

AN APPLE A DAY KEEPS EXCESS FAT AWAY

If your child has a problem with overeating at mealtime, try offering an apple twenty minutes before lunch or dinner. Apples, which are high in fiber and low in calories, satisfy just enough to curb overeating yet do not dampen the appetite so much that your child misses out on a healthy meal.

---

fat calories. Of course, high-fiber foods are usually low in fat themselves.

Fiber helps you feel good after eating. Fiber slows the absorption of sugar from the intestines. This means your blood sugar level is steadier after a high-fiber meal. Fiber lowers the meal's glycemic load, the measure of how fast a food triggers the blood insulin cycle.

Fiber is good for the gut. People who eat fiber-rich diets have a lower incidence of intestinal problems, from colitis to colon cancer. Fiber acts like a broom, gathering up possibly toxic waste products and sweeping them through the intestines. This cuts down on the amount of time that the lining of the bowel walls is exposed to potential disease-causing substances. Fiber sweeps out waste before it can do any harm. Fiber also fosters good gut health by promoting the growth of friendly bacteria in the colon that help with the absorption of certain vitamins and essential fats. Fiber, along with plenty of water, also prevents constipation, a common problem for many children.

Fiber is heart healthy. Fiber lowers levels of bad cholesterol (LDL) without lowering good cholesterol (HDL) levels. As it travels through the intestines, fiber absorbs water, forming a gluey gel that picks up some of the cholesterol from food and carries it out of the body. Research shows that increasing the amount of fiber in your diet decreases the incidence of cardiovascular disease, intestinal cancers, and diabetes.

How much fiber should your family eat? Most adults and children consume only about half the fiber they need. Here are goals for adding fiber to your family's diet:

- Adults: 25–35 grams of fiber daily.
- Children: the child's age plus at least 10 grams daily. A five-year-old should eat at least 15 grams of fiber a day.
- The recommended amount of fiber is 14 grams for each 1,000 calories consumed. If you eat 2,000 calories in a day, you should consume at least 28 grams of fiber.

Five Fiber-Eating Tips

The standard American diet (SAD) of meat, dairy, and white bread is ridiculously low in fiber. The modern SAD shopper bypasses the areas in the supermarket that contain the most fiber, fills her basket in the fiberless aisles, and then heads for the laxative shelf to pick up fiber in a jar. It's better to get your fiber from the original sources — foods that come from plants. Enjoy these five fiber-eating tips:

1. Fill up with fiber first. Eat fiber-rich foods such as a big salad at the beginning of a meal. You will fill your stomach and feel less inclined to overeat any high-calorie foods that follow. Most high-fiber foods are "free foods," meaning you can eat all you want without worrying about taking in too many calories. Good news for overeaters!

2. Eat "whole" foods. To get more fiber in your child's diet, encourage her to eat every edible part of the fruit or vegetable. The peel on apples and the white pith on oranges are rich sources of fiber, as are potato skins. Fresh fruits have more fiber than canned fruits because much of the fiber is in the peel, which is usually removed in processing. Whole fruits are better than fruit juices, and nectars are usually more fiber-rich than juices. Instead of fiber-poor white bread, eat breads made with whole wheat flour. Choose whole-grain cereals that contain wheat bran, oat bran, wheat germ, or barley. Instead of white rice, eat brown or wild rice. Cut back on refined foods, even if they claim to be enriched. The fiber that was originally there is virtually absent from many refined or enriched foods.

Enjoy the ABC's of favorite fiber foods:

A: apples, avocados, artichokes
B: beans, bran, barley, berries
C: cereals (those with at least 3–5 grams of fiber per serving)
S: salads and raw vegetables

3. Eat fiber from a variety of sources. There are two types of fiber. Soluble fiber, the type found in beans, peas, bran, barley, and fruit pectin acts like a sponge, absorbing water and turning food into a soft gel that moves easily through the intestines. Insoluble fiber is the stringy stuff from leaves, peels, skins, and the coverings of seeds and grains. This type of fiber acts like a broom to sweep intestinal contents along. Your body needs both types of fiber, so be sure to eat grains and legumes as well as fresh fruits and veggies.

4. Drink lots of water with your fiber. Fiber soaks up water in the gut. When you increase the fiber in your diet, be sure to drink more water to keep that fiber moving through your intestines. Otherwise, adding fiber to your diet may actually contribute to constipation rather than prevent it. As a general guide, your child needs to drink ¾ to 1 ounce of fluids per pound of body weight. So a 40-pound child should drink at least 30 to 40 ounces per day.

5. Increase fiber gradually. A sudden increase in the amount of fiber you eat can catch your gut off guard. Your body won't be up to the challenge of digesting this bulky stuff, and you will feel bloated and gassy. For a more comfortable gut feeling, add fiber to your diet gradually and eat fiber-rich foods throughout the day, not just at one meal. Each week increase the amount of fiber in your daily diet by about 5 grams for adults and 1 or 2 grams for children. Experiment with different types and different amounts of fiber-rich foods until you find what works best for you.

Getting Kids to Eat More Fiber

Kids get constipated, and parents complain to pediatricians. It's not easy to persuade children to eat more of the foods that will help them move their bowels, but it's possible if you make fiber look like fun. Here are some ways to help your kids enjoy eating high-fiber foods:

Try a daily high-fiber yogurt smoothie. Add a couple handfuls of fresh or frozen fruit (choose from strawberries, bananas, papayas, mangoes, blueberries, and pears) and 2 tablespoons of ground flaxseeds to a cup of yogurt and whirl it around in the blender. (For a recipe, see page 298.)

Serve dried fruits. Apricots, figs, prunes, dates, raisins, and cranberries are all high in fiber.

Be a bean freak. Beans (e.g., black, kidney) are a rich source of fiber. You can add them to many foods that kids already eat: salads, soups, burritos, and chili.

BEST FIBER FOODS

Fiber Food	Serving Size	Fiber (in grams)
Psyllium husks	2 tbsp. (1 ounce)	16
High-fiber cereals	1 ounce (½ cup)	10–14
Flaxseed meal	¼ cup	8
Barley	½ cup	8
Artichokes	½ medium	8
Kidney beans	½ cup	7.3
Chickpeas (garbanzo beans)	½ cup	7
Figs (dried)	3 medium	5.3
Navy beans	½ cup	6
Prunes	3 medium	3
Oat bran	¼ cup	4
Apples (with skin)	1 medium	3.5
Pita bread (whole wheat)	1 piece	5
Corn	1 ear	5
Lima beans	½ cup	4.5
Avocados	½	4
Lentils (such as in soup)	½ cup	3.7
Peas	½ cup	3.6
Spaghetti (whole wheat)	1 cup	3.9
Pears	1 medium	3.2
Sweet potatoes	½ cup	3
Oranges (with membrane)	1	2.6
Spinach	½ cup	2.5
Potatoes (with skin)	1 medium	2.5
Bananas	1 medium	2.4
Broccoli	½ cup	2.3
Popcorn (homemade)	2 cups	2.0
Blueberries	½ cup	2.0
Grapefruit (with membrane)	½	1.6
Apricots (dried)	5 halves	1.4
Bread (whole wheat)	1 slice	1.4

Dip it. Smash or purée beans to make high-fiber dips. Hummus, made from chickpeas, is nutritious, fiber-rich, and fun to spread on bread, crackers, or raw veggies.

Choose a high-fiber cereal. Most kids love cereal, so steer your children to high-fiber choices, ones that have at least 3 grams of fiber per serving. Or boost the fiber content of their favorite cereal by mixing in a tablespoon of flaxseed meal.

Pick the greenest greens. Spinach and romaine lettuce offer far more fiber than iceberg lettuce. Use these darker greens in salads so that your kids get the maximum amount of nutrients from every bite they take.

Don't skimp on the skin. Serve fruits such as apples and pears with their skins on, cut into easy-to-eat wedges or slices. (Buy organic fruits to avoid pesticides in the peels.) If you serve homemade french fries, or, even better, sweet potato fries, leave the skins on. Encourage your children to eat whole fruit rather than just drinking fruit juice. When you do serve fruit juice, choose fruit nectars, since these thicker juices include the fruit pulp and have a bit more fiber than more refined juices.

SERVE SUPER SNACKS THAT SATISFY

Remember that grazing is good for you only if you graze on healthy food. When your children are choosing snacks, steer them toward grow foods. Send grow-food snacks along with your child to school and day care. Snacks that are good for grazing leave kids feeling satisfied but not too full. Here are some guidelines for healthy snacking and grazing:

Pack protein in every snack. Protein-rich foods trigger satiety better than any other food, so they curb overeating. Eating protein as part of every meal and snack stabilizes blood sugar. Eating protein-rich foods is the key to making grazing work for you.

Figure in fiber. As we've mentioned repeatedly throughout this book, fiber is filling without being fattening. Fiber-rich foods fill the tummy and slow down the absorption of carbs, so blood sugar and insulin levels stay steady.

Waterlog the snacks. Foods with a high water content, such as fruits and soup, give more volume without a lot of calories.

Always partner carbs with protein, fiber, and perhaps some healthy fat. Never eat a carb-only snack. Carb-only foods (also known as empty carbs) are not filling or satisfying. They are digested quickly, so that blood sugar levels rise and fall rapidly, triggering hunger and another urgent snack attack. In the satiety pecking order, protein comes first, fats second, fiber-rich carbs third, and empty carbs a distant fourth. Empty carbs also make your brain sleepy.

Allow frequent snacking. The younger the child, the more frequent the snacks. Toddlers may need to nibble on healthy food every two hours; preschoolers and school-age children may enjoy three snacks a day, at midmorning, midafternoon, and before bed.

Structure the snacks. It is unusual for a child to overeat nutritious foods. If a child's only choices are grow foods because you refuse to buy the other stuff, you probably don't have to worry about when and how often kids eat. Prepare a nibble tray of healthy snacks and leave it on the kitchen table. Most kids can be trusted to snack appropriately throughout the day, but some children cannot handle free access to the pantry and refrigerator. Or they may get so involved in play that they forget to eat. You may find that scheduling regular snacks works better for your family. That late-afternoon snack may be essential to keeping the peace while you prepare dinner.

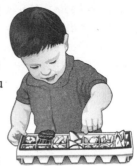

Avoid mindless snacking. Discourage children from munching in front of the television or while playing video games. Kids tend to overeat when their mind isn't on what they are eating. Instead of handing the whole box of crackers to your child, pour a serving into a bowl and then put the box away.

KISMIF — keep it small, make it filling. A healthy-size snack is about the size of the eater's fist. If you're eating nutrient-dense foods such as nuts, the amount that fits in the palm of your hand should be enough to satisfy. Snacks for school-age children should contain between 100 and 200 calories. Choose snacks that are quick and easy to prepare. Let your children pick out some

---

NIBBLING ON NUTS

During the writing of this book, I (Dr. Bill) had the privilege of serving as a volunteer doctor in the area of Indonesia hit by the tsunami. Our medical clinic was on the devastated island of Nias in the middle of the jungle. My diet for a week was nuts, a small can of salmon a day, and fruit I could pick off local trees. I snacked on nuts all day. Even though that week was one of the most exhausting I have experienced, I enjoyed a good gut feeling and had lots of physical and mental energy, which I attribute — at least partially — to nibbling on nuts.

favorites from the Super Snack List on the facing page when you're preparing your grocery list.

Go nuts. Our top pick for a nutritious snack food is nuts. Besides being nutrient dense — full of healthy fats, protein, fiber, vitamins, and minerals — nuts are a great fill-up food. A handful of raw nuts (around 150 calories) is a just-right snack.

THE SIPPING SOLUTION

"Sipping" is a term we use for liquid grazing. I (Dr. Bill) discovered this way of eating, or rather, drinking, while I was undergoing radiation and chemotherapy for colon cancer. It was difficult for me to eat solid foods, so for six months I lived mainly on high-fiber, nutrient-dense smoothies. Every morning I would make a smoothie that totaled about 1,300 calories, and sip on it throughout the day. After a few weeks, I noticed a good gut feeling (which is unusual during cancer treatment!). I was never hungry, never too full, but always satisfied. I was experiencing all the biochemical perks of grazing from sipping this nutritious liquid. I was surprised because I had always believed that liquid foods were not as satisfying as solid ones. I got so used to the good gut feeling and mental alertness I felt from sipping on this nutritious smoothie all day that I still continue this way of eating at least five days a week. The smoothie is my breakfast, lunch, and snacks, followed by a regular meal in the evening. On a day when I need more calories for extra energy, I add 1 or 2 tablespoons of peanut butter to the smoothie or nibble on nuts, too. If you want to feel the perks of being in biochemical balance, try this sipping solution. (See Dr. Bill's smoothie recipe, page 298.)

Super Snack List

Here's a list of good foods for grazing. These are super snacks, ones that partner carbs with protein, fiber, and/or healthy fats. Your children will find lots to like on this list.

- carrot sticks dipped in hummus
- apple slices dipped in peanut butter
- whole-grain cereal with yogurt
- edamame (fresh, cooked soybeans)
- string cheese and a piece of fruit
- cottage cheese and fruit
- a handful of raw nuts or trail mix
- pita bread spread with hummus
- rice cake with peanut butter and banana
- Parmesan cheese melted on a slice of whole-grain bread
- blueberries in yogurt
- popcorn (homemade air popped)
- celery sticks with peanut butter
- cherry tomatoes with cheese cubes
- fruit-and-yogurt smoothie
- hard-boiled egg
- bean dip and veggie sticks
- any fruit
- whole-grain, preferably homemade muffins
- homemade oatmeal-raisin cookies (see recipe, page 304)
- cut-up vegetables with salsa and corn chips

7

Eleven Ways to Feed Growing Brains

The brain grows rapidly in the first five years of a child's life. It triples in volume during the first two years and reaches 90 percent of its adult size by five years of age. Rapid growth uses energy, and in fact, infants use up to 60 percent of the energy they get from food for brain growth. Even in older children, teens, and adults, the brain uses about 25 percent of total food energy, though the brain itself makes up only about 2 percent of a child's body weight. Above all other organs, the brain is most affected — for better or worse — by what we eat.

One day we were visiting friends, and the mother complained about her child's behavior, "I don't know what's gotten into him . . ." After spending some time in their kitchen, I realized what had gotten into him. Junk food!

HOW SMART FOODS BUILD SMART BRAINS

The brain is composed of trillions of specialized cells called neurons. The cells contain a number of different structures, each of which has an important job to do. All of these structures are made out of raw materials that come from the food you eat. They also depend on high-quality nutrition for the energy you need in order to think and learn.

DOES YOUR CHILD HAVE N.D.D.?

Oftentimes parents bring their child to me for consultation on learning or behavioral problems at school. They typically open their concern with, "We and our child's teacher believe he has A.D.D. . . ." After taking a nutritional history, I often reply, "Your child doesn't have A.D.D., he has N.D.D." Obviously, they look surprised. They don't know what N.D.D. is, but it doesn't sound like something they want their child to have. I go on to explain that what I mean by N.D.D. is a nutrition deficit disorder. In my experience, many children described as having A.D.D. lose this tag once their N.D.D. is treated. You will now learn how to do this.

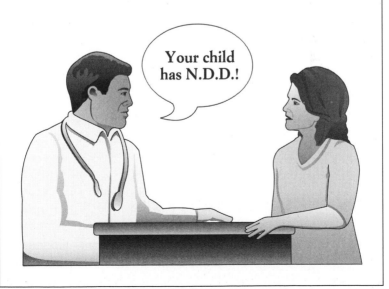

Let's look into your child's growing brain to see how the food your child eats affects brain cells and the way they function.

- The *cell membrane* is a filter that allows good stuff into the cell while keeping bad stuff out. Certain nutrients like omega-3 fats and the antioxidants in fruits and vegetables form the structural and functional components of the cell membrane.

- The *cell itself* is really a microscopic energy-processing factory. Brain cells turn the glucose in the blood into energy to manufacture substances that help the brain think and repair itself.

- The *axon* is like an electrical wire projecting from the neuron. Electrical impulses travel down the axon, causing it to release *neurotransmitters,* substances that carry messages across the gap between cells to receptor sites on the *dendrites* of the next neuron. A fatty sheath called *myelin* covers the axon, like insulation around an electrical wire, and speeds the transmission of electrical impulses. The more omega-3 fats in the diet, the better the quality of this insulation, and the more efficiently neurons can communicate.

- The *synapses* are the gaps between the cells. The *dendrites* are fingerlike projections from the end of the nerve cell that attempt to connect with other brain cells across the synapse. Brain researchers estimate that the growing brain of a child can make a couple million connections between neurons every second. It's the connections between neurons that account for most of the brain growth in the early years. Building connections — pathways — between neurons is how the brain makes sense of information coming in, how it remembers things, and how it signals muscles to react and move. Growing more connections makes the brain smarter.

Feeding the brain is like feeding your computer — garbage in equals garbage out. These brain cell structures are affected by what you eat and when you eat it. Smart eating means choosing the right fats and carbs and combining them

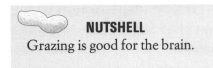

NUTSHELL

Grazing is good for the brain.

with protein so that your brain grows healthy cells, makes healthy connections, and operates calmly and efficiently.

1. FEED YOUR FAMILY SMART FATS

Since the brain is 60 percent fat, it stands to reason that growing brains need high-quality fats. Smart fats make the brain grow and perform better. Smart fats, as you learned in chapter 4, are the omega-3 fatty acids that are found in especially high amounts in seafood. Omega-3 fats are also found in some plants (e.g., flaxseed oil, canola oil, nuts, and seeds), but the omega-3 fats found in plants have to be converted from shorter-chain fatty acids to longer ones before they can be used in the brain. Seafood is the most direct source of long-chain omega 3's.

Eat fish, be smart. Oceans of recent research show that omega-3 fats make brains healthier, especially the brains of young kids and older adults. Researchers believe that the high levels of omega-3 fats in breast milk help to explain the differences in IQ between children who received human milk in infancy and those who did not. The body uses omega-3 fats to make cell membranes. Omega-3 fats are also needed to make myelin, the insulation around nerves, and to help neurotransmitters function at the optimal levels. Omega-3 fats are known as essential fatty acids, because it is essential to get these fatty acids from food. Other types of fats can be manufactured in the body, but the body cannot make essential fatty acids. That is why it is important for growing brains to get adequate amounts of these smart fats from food. If there are not enough "smart" fats available to make brain cells and other key substances, the body uses lesser-quality fats and produces lesser-quality cells. The "dumb" fats (known as replacement fatty acids), the kind that come from the trans fats in hydrogenated oils, clog the receptors in the cell membrane, and the brain cell does not function as well.

Neurotransmitters, the biochemical messengers that carry information from one brain cell to another, fit into receptors on cell membranes like a key fits into a lock. The keys and the locks must match. If the cell membrane is composed of the right fats, the locks and keys match. But if the receptors are clogged with the

---

ENJOY A MEDICINE MEAL

I (Dr. Bill) experienced a vivid demonstration of the brain-boosting effects of seafood when I was on a speaking tour of Japan in 2001. Before one of the talks, our Japanese hosts told Martha and me that they were going to take us out for a "medicine meal." They explained that this meal was a century-old tradition in which a visiting professor is served a special meal before he gives a lecture. Normally I don't eat much before giving a talk, but it would have been rude to refuse the invitation. So we went out to lunch, where we were presented with a tray holding fifteen little dishes that we had never seen before. When our interpreter checked the name of each food with his pocket translator, the results were all "edible seafoods." That medicine meal was a combination of many different fish and sea plants. An hour after I ate, my brain was amazingly alert. I also had what I call a "good gut" feeling, neither hungry nor full. That good feeling in my brain and gut stayed with me for at least four hours, confirming my belief in the brain-boosting effects of omega-3 fats in seafood. I gave one of my best talks ever!

wrong fats, the neurotransmitter keys won't fit, and brain-cell function suffers. Omega-3 fats keep the receptors open so the neurotransmitters fit and the brain can function optimally.

Eat fish, be happy. In the last ten years, pediatricians and psychiatrists have increasingly prescribed a wider variety of mood-altering and behavior-changing medications for kids. This is partly because parents and professionals have become more aware that many children and teens struggle with depression and that they can benefit from treatment. But we wonder if the SAD diet could be another factor in the increasing incidence of mood and behavior disorders in both kids and adults.

One of the most exciting developments in the concept of food as medicine in the past few years has been the use of diets high in omega-3 fats to stabilize moods. Mood and anxiety disorders are accompanied by biochemical imbalances in the brain and are triggered by difficult life events. Antidepressant or anti-anxiety medications alter brain chemistry in ways that may relieve symptoms of sadness or excessive worry. And now research is showing that omega-3 fats also have mood-elevating and calming effects on the brain, boosting levels of "happy neurotransmitters." Consider the following:

- In one study, people whose diets were high in omega-6 fats and low in omega-3 fats (the typical SAD diet) had a higher incidence of depression.

- In another study, depressed people who ate salmon every day showed greater improvement than people treated with standard antidepressant medications.

- Postpartum depression was found to be less severe in women who ate more seafood.

- People with bipolar disorder who took fish oil capsules in combination with standard medications showed greater mood stabilization.

Omega-3 fats are important to the structure and function of neurotransmitters in the brain, so it makes sense that a diet high in these "happy fats" helps the brain stay happy.

Eat fish, learn and behave better. In order for kids to learn, they have to be able to concentrate. Studies show that omega-3 fats help the brain pay attention and make connections. Researchers at Purdue University found that boys with A.D.H.D. (Attention Deficit Hyperactivity Disorder) had lower levels of omega-3 fats, especially DHA, the main omega-3 fat found in fish. The boys with the most abnormal behavior had the lowest levels of DHA. School-age children with the highest levels of omega-3 fatty acids in their blood had the fewest learning problems. In addition, students who were given DHA supplements prior to exams showed less hostility and aggression during this time of stress.

Smart fats for teen brains. Since both brains and bodies go through another growth spurt in the teen years, adolescence is another stage when eating smart fats is important. Yet, just at the stage when teens need smart fats, they tend to eat more dumb fats. Time pressures and the availability of fast food cause most teens to wind up with a diet high in unhealthy fats, such as the saturated, artery-clogging fats in fatty meat and the hydrogenated fats in doughnuts and french fries. And just at the stage when they need a diet high in smart fats, many teens go on a low-fat diet.

NUTSHELL
Teen brains need more fish and fewer fries.

SCIENCE SAYS: SEAFOOD IS SMART FOOD

Here's more on what science says about how a diet rich in omega-3 fats can improve learning and behavior:

- Infants who receive infant formula that contains DHA, an omega-3 fatty acid, have higher IQs and better visual acuity than those receiving regular formula. Human milk contains high levels of omega-3 fats, a clue that these fats are important to infant development. Before 2002, formulas made in America did not contain DHA.

- Populations whose diet is high in omega-3 fats have a lower incidence of degenerative diseases of the central nervous system, such as multiple sclerosis.

- Experimental animals whose diets are low in the brain-building omega-3 fat DHA have been found to have smaller brains and delayed brain development.

- Animal studies show that omega-3 fats increase levels of dopamine and the number of dopamine receptors in the brain. Dopamine is a neurotransmitter that helps the brain stay alert.

- A diet high in omega-3 fats helps not only the very young but the very old, too. Research shows that senior citizens who eat more fish are less likely to develop dementia.

2. FEED YOUR FAMILY SMART CARBS AND PROTEINS

Around 50 percent of the energy from the carbohydrates children eat goes to fueling their growing brains. Muscles can store glucose, the body's main fuel, extracted from digested carbs. But the brain can't store much glucose. It depends on a steady supply of glucose in the bloodstream. If the blood sugar dips too low, brain function can deteriorate within minutes. The brain is very selective about the carbs it craves, and it prefers that you eat the right carbs with the right partners at the right time. (For an explanation of how healthy carbs behave well in the brain and junk carbs don't, read chapter 3.) If brain cells could comment on the best ways to give them the carbs they need, here's what they would request:

Partner carbs with fiber and protein. As you learned in chapter 3, the brain prefers carbs that are naturally packaged with protein and fiber. These two partners slow the digestive process and steady the rate at which glucose enters the blood. Without protein or fiber in a food, the carbs are digested quickly and rush into the bloodstream so fast that they cause a sugar high followed by a sugar low, as the body releases a large amount of insulin to handle the sugar. Unstable blood sugar levels lead to unstable brain chemistry, which makes it hard for kids to pay attention and control their behavior. The sudden drop in blood sugar that follows a sugar high also triggers the release of stress hormones. This is why kids' behavior can deteriorate rapidly after snacks of sweetened beverages and other junky carbs. They get jumpy and irritable, and eventually, because of high serotonin levels triggered by a carb overdose, they get sleepy. Yet, eating a carb-rich snack or meal that also contains fiber and protein and some healthy fats leaves children feeling relaxed and alert. The slow but steady release of glucose into the blood gives the brain the energy it needs without causing jolts of jitteriness or the foggy feeling that leads to poor attention and learning.

Graze on good carbs. Kids and adults don't think well when they're hungry. Frequent mini-meals throughout the day are good for the brain. When you graze on the right foods, you never get too hungry and never feel too full. The brain gets a steady supply of fuel from high-fiber carbs, proteins, and healthy fats. We have found that trail mix made with nuts and dried fruit (see recipe, page 302) is one of the best grazing foods. Your brain's advice on snacks would be "Go nuts!"

Eat protein for brain power. High-protein foods perk up the brain by increasing levels of two "alertness" neurotransmitters, dopamine and norepinephrine. A high-protein meal really is a "power breakfast" or a "power lunch," because it helps kids perform at their best at school and parents perform at their best at work. Protein also contains the amino acid tryptophan, which is one of the building blocks of serotonin. Steady levels of serotonin contribute to a steady feeling of well-being. In our practice we frequently see improvements in a child's mood and learning abilities when we suggest these two changes in their diet:

- Add more protein to each meal and snack.
- Avoid fiberless carbs (e.g., candy and soda). Instead, choose the fiber-filled carbs in fruits, vegetables, nuts, and whole grains.

3. FEED THE BRAIN SMART FOODS AT THE RIGHT TIMES OF THE DAY

Have you ever had to go back to work after enjoying a big meal? Or dozed off during the after-dinner speeches at a fancy banquet? Too many carbs and fats will put the brain to sleep. You may welcome this drowsy feeling at bedtime, but it won't help your performance at work or your child's performance at school. Brains function better on smaller amounts of food, in just the right proportions of carbs, fats, and proteins, eaten throughout the day.

BEST SNACKS FOR PRESCHOOL AND KINDERGARTEN

It's especially important for school snacks to be nutritious. The snacks listed below have the right combination of carbs, protein, and fat to keep kids alert, satisfied, and able to learn:

- a handful of raw nuts or trail mix
- peanut butter on apple slices
- hard-boiled egg
- yogurt, plain, with nuts and fresh fruit or granola
- homemade oatmeal-raisin cookies (see recipe, page 304) and a cup of low-fat milk
- edamame (fresh, cooked soybeans)

For more snack suggestions, see page 166.

You can use what you know about the effects of food on the brain to give your children a smart nutritional start in the morning and a soothing evening meal before bedtime. Some combinations of nutrients are neuron turn-ons that perk up the brain; others are neuron wind-downs that have a calming or sedative effect. Here are some suggestions:

Breakfast. Since proteins perk up the brain, send your kids off to school with a high-protein, healthy-carb, and healthy-fat breakfast, such as whole-grain cereal and yogurt. (For examples of brainy breakfasts, see page 191.)

Lunch. To continue to run, jump, play, and learn all afternoon, kids should eat another high-protein, healthy-carb, and healthy-fat meal for lunch, such as a super salad: spinach, hard-boiled egg or tuna, raisins, and walnuts. Skip the dessert and heavy fried foods at lunch. These foods make children sleepy. (See page 287 for suggestions for healthy school meals.)

Dinner. The evening meal could have more carbs and less protein, along with a moderate amount of healthy fat. Pasta is better served for dinner than for lunch. And now would be the time to enjoy the dessert you didn't serve at lunchtime.

You can see that the combination of nutrients at dinner is the reverse of breakfast and lunch — fewer carbs and more protein during the day, more carbs and less protein in the evening. These breakfast and lunch combinations should perk up the brain, and the dinner combinations relax it. Our culture tends to do the opposite. Unless you want your young student to need a siesta, skip the high-carb, high-calorie, high-fat foods at midday.

NUTSHELL
Shorten the space between feedings and you are less likely to have spacey kids.

4. FIGURE OUT YOUR CHILD'S MOOD FOODS

Foods can change a child's mood. This is more noticeable in some children than in others. Some kids are exquisitely sensitive to sugar. Their mothers report, "Her behavior completely deteriorates after a can of soda or a candy bar." Some parents and teachers report that children's attention span and behavior at school is compromised by a junk-food breakfast or lunch. Other very observant parents notice connections between their child's behavior and various sweeteners and chemical additives in the foods they eat. Not every child's behavior and ability to learn seems to be noticeably affected by diet. Here are some tips to help you figure out if a food-mood connection is influencing your child's behavior:

Watch for a change in behavior following a change in eating. If you're a 90/10 family (90 percent healthy foods and 10 percent junk foods), you may notice junky behavior when you let down your usual eating habits and allow your kids more junk-food treats, perhaps during a holiday or on a vacation. Help your child recognize that his sluggishness is a result of a syrupy, high-carb breakfast or a lunch of breaded chicken strips and french fries. Remember that part of shaping young tastes is teaching children to pay attention to their own food-mood connections.

Observe changes in behavior and learning after de-junking the diet. Suppose your child is having a learning or behavior problem at school. Change what the child eats for breakfast. Take away the junk carbs and add fiber and protein, plus some healthy fat. After a couple of weeks of the new morning menus (see suggestions, page 191), ask your child's teachers if they notice any difference. Pack a nutritious lunch instead of letting your child purchase junk food at school, and ask the teachers and your child if they notice any difference. Oftentimes just replacing junk carbs with protein can make a big difference in the behavior of children who have been either hyper or groggy during the school day.

Offer sweet treats with an otherwise healthy meal. When kids ask for sweet treats (and they will, no matter how much you discourage this), and you want to say yes now and then, be sure they eat these treats as part of a high-protein, healthy-carb, and healthy-fat meal. Protein, fiber, and fat help to level out the roller-coaster effect of eating sweets. For many children the food-mood connection is dose related: small amounts of sweets have little effect, but large amounts bother them. They may get hyper or "fog out" after downing a 12-ounce cola on an empty stomach, yet the sugar in the cola doesn't seem to bother them if they drink it with an otherwise healthy meal.

Try keeping a food record of what your child eats. Don't make an issue of his food choices, or he might be tempted to sneak the foods he should avoid.

SAMPLE FOOD-MOOD CONNECTION RECORD

When my child eats/drinks . . .   **He feels/acts . . .**

a lot of artificially colored and   he can't sit still or think
sugary punch . . .   straight for the rest of the day

_____   _____

_____   _____

_____   _____

Enlist your child's cooperation. From your own observations and from periodically quizzing your child, try to figure out which foods make him feel happy and comfortable and which ones make him feel restless and irritable. You could even make a list with your child, dividing foods into "happy foods" and "sad foods." Our list on the next page is an example. Once children become more aware of their own personal food-mood connections, they are more likely to avoid foods that make them feel bad.

5. EAT GREEN

Don't forget your folate. Folate (also called folic acid) is vital for growing healthy brain cells and preserving neurotransmitter

---

HAPPY VS. SAD FOODS

Happy Foods	Sad Foods or Fidget Foods
• blueberries	• bakery "bads"
• eggs	• candy bars
• fruits	• french fries
• high-fiber cereals	• gelatin desserts
• nut butters	• juice drinks
• oatmeal-raisin cookie	• junk cereals
• salads	• sodas
• salmon	
• yogurt	

---

function. Best sources of folic acid are green, leafy vegetables, such as collard greens, bok choy, and spinach, and also asparagus. Other rich sources are lentils, chickpeas, kidney beans, artichokes, avocados, and cereals fortified with folic acid.

6. EAT BLUE

Blueberries are a great brain food. The deep blue skin of the blueberry is full of flavonoids, especially anthocyanin, an antioxidant that helps keep both growing and aging brains healthy. One study, dubbed the "Blueberry Rats Study," compared a control group of rats with another group, which were fed blueberries. The blueberry rats showed improved balance and motor coordination. The blueberry diet also reversed the effects of mental aging in these rats and made them act more youthful. Neuroscientists believe that one of the main benefits of eating foods such as green greens and deep-colored berries, which contain high levels of antioxidants, is the effect on the blood-brain barrier — a membranelike tissue only a cell-layer thick that keeps toxic substances from entering the brain and causing harm. The researchers behind the Blueberry Rats Study also concluded that nutrients in blueberries improved the way neurons talk to each

---

BERRY GOOD BRAINS

We rank berries, especially blueberries, as one of our top twelve health foods for many good reasons. Blueberries are a prime example of the color principle: The deeper the color of the food, the better it is for you. Colorful berries are full of phytonutrients. This is especially so for blueberry skins, which contain powerful antioxidants called anthocyanins. In a study that tested antioxidant levels in forty fruits and vegetables, blueberries received the top prize. Here are some more good things about blueberries:

- Blueberries contain an anticancer antioxidant called elegiac acid.

- Blueberries exert an anti-inflammatory effect, protecting the tissues of the brain, muscle, and digestive tract from excessive wear and tear.

- Blueberries contain substances that promote vasodilatation — they open up blood vessels so that blood can flow more freely. Blueberries also help prevent blood clots. So blueberries, besides claiming the title of "brain berry," also deserve to be known as a "heart berry."

- Blueberries improve motor skill performance.

- Blueberries, like cranberries, have antibacterial properties that decrease the risk of urinary tract infections.

other. Another animal study showed that blueberries in the diet increased the concentration of the neurotransmitter dopamine in the animals' brains. These are all good reasons for dubbing blueberries the "brain berry." Try adding blueberries to muffins, cereals (a couple tablespoons of blueberries is all the sweetener a cereal needs), pancakes, and smoothies. Eating blue can keep you from feeling blue.

7. DON'T FORGET YOUR PHYTOS

Because the brain burns so much energy, it also produces "exhaust," metabolic by-products called free radicals. These cause oxidation, damage to body tissues similar to rust on iron. Antioxidants fight this damage so that cells stay healthy. Higher amounts of antioxidants in the diet are associated with lower risks of cancer, heart disease, and degenerative diseases of the brain. Uncontrolled oxidation is thought to be the primary cause of premature aging in the brain and for the decline in brain function as people age. Antioxidants are phytonutrients — nutrients that come from plants. When you serve your family a wide variety of plant foods, you put many kinds of antioxidants to work in those growing bodies and keep growing brains in good repair. As pediatricians, we are concerned that children are aging too quickly. (For our list of top phytos, see page 197.)

8. MIND YOUR MINERALS

Minerals that are the most important for optimal brain function are iron, calcium, and zinc. (See Vitamin and Mineral Supplements, pages 262 to 273, for rich food sources of these nutrients and how they help brain function.)

9. EXCLUDE EXCITOTOXINS

"Excitotoxin" may be a term that is new to you. Excitotoxins are food additives such as aspartame and MSG, aka hydrolyzed vegetable protein, that can alter the chemistry of the brain. Studies in experimental animals show that some of the chemicals that are routinely added to processed food can damage the parts of the brain cell called the mitochondria (the energy center of the cell) and also throw neurotransmitter activity out of balance. Whether this same neurochemical upset occurs in humans is controversial. Some medical scientists believe that excitotoxins play a role in the development of many different neurological diseases, including Parkinson's disease, seizures, and Alzheimer's disease. These additives serve no useful nutritional function, so why take the chance? It's best to avoid food additives, especially aspartame and MSG, as much as you can.

The rapidly growing brains of children may be even more vul-

BRAIN FOODS

Here are the best and worst foods for the brain.

Smart Foods	"Dumb" Foods
• blueberries	• excitotoxins, e.g., MSG, aspartame, food colorings, and preservatives
• nuts	
• salmon	• fiber-poor carbs
• spinach	• hydrogenated oils
	• "liquid candy" — sweetened beverages

nerable to excitotoxins than adult brains are, and some children may show more dramatic effects than others. According to neurosurgeon Russell Blaylock, author of *Excitotoxins: The Taste That Kills,* a child's brain is four times more sensitive to excitotoxins than the adult brain is. Here's where your food-mood observations help. Some children, and some adults, experience severe headaches and mood swings following the ingestion of aspartame or MSG, for example. Some notice only that they feel "weird" or can't focus as well. Remember the "pure" kids you met in chapter 1? Their "pure parents" wisely scrutinize food labels for any ingredients that sound like they came from a chemistry lab rather than from nature, and they ban these foods from their homes. Their kids are healthier as a result.

BAN THE "BAD WORDS"

For the brain health of your family, avoid processed foods that contain these additives:

- aspartame
- MSG
- hydrolyzed vegetable protein
- BHT and other preservatives

- red #40
- blue #1
- yellow #6
- any other color-number combo

The body, in its wisdom, protects growing brains and tissues from some toxins in the diet. The blood-brain barrier keeps many potentially harmful substances from crossing over into the brain. Yet it cannot protect brain cells from every potential threat. While the brain can probably safely process some of the chemical substances added to foods, it's best to avoid excessive amounts.

10. MOVE!

Physical exercise is good for brains as well as bodies, so get your kids up and moving. Consider movement another brain food. Here are three ways that exercise makes brains smarter:

Exercise improves blood flow to the brain. Improving blood flow to any organ, especially the brain, is like watering and fertilizing a garden. More blood means more nutrients. When you move your muscles, especially the large muscles in your arms and legs, which you use in vigorous exercise, your heart works harder to pump blood through your veins and arteries.

While writing this book, I (Dr. Bill) had the opportunity to have lunch with Dr. Lou Ignarro, who in 1998 won the Nobel Prize in Physiology or Medicine for the discovery of how nitric oxide (which I call the body's "natural health juice") affects blood vessels. Here's how Dr. Lou explained it to me: "When you exercise, in response to the faster movement of blood through the blood vessels, the lining of the vessels secretes a natural substance called nitric oxide, or NO for short. NO makes blood vessels dilate. They open up so that more blood can flow, and this brings more nutrients to the brain and to the rest of the body."

After listening to Lou, I responded, "So exercising is like teaching the body and brain to muster up its own internal medicine."

"You got it!" he replied.

Exercise stimulates nerve growth factors (NGF). Nerve growth factors help the body grow and repair nerve cells. The increased blood flow from movement stimulates the release of NGF, keeping the brain in good operating condition.

Exercise releases happy hormones. Increasing blood flow to the brain stimulates the release of mood-elevating hormones. The same neurochemicals that relax the blood vessels relax the brain. This helps both body and brain cope with stress. Exercise helps the body muster up its own internal medicine to combat depression and worry. For many people, exercise is a healthier alternative to mood-altering medications.

11. BEGIN THE DAY WITH A BRAINY BREAKFAST

Breakfast is just what the word says: the breaking of a fast, one that is ten to twelve hours long for many children. During the night the gut rests and the body's chemistry settles down. Unless you've upset your metabolism by indulging in a junk-food snack before going to bed, your body should enjoy a steady state of biochemical balance during sleep. By making wise choices about the foods you eat to break your overnight fast, you can keep this feeling of biochemical balance going through to lunchtime.

Adults as well as children need a healthy breakfast. Many children skip breakfast or eat junk carbs in the morning because that's what they see their parents do. A quick cup of coffee and a doughnut grabbed on the run may satisfy your hunger for a short time, but it won't give your brain the steady supply of fuel it needs to work hard all morning. Make breakfast a family priority. Both you and your children will benefit.

Three Reasons Why Breakfast Is the Most Important Meal

Sending your child off to school without breakfast is like taking your car out on the road with a near-empty gas tank. Simply put, children need fuel. Here's why breakfast is the most important meal of the day for school-age kids.

1. Breakfast builds brighter brains. Eating a healthy breakfast perks up a child's metabolism, which perks up the brain and gets it ready for learning. The brain needs a steady supply of good fuel to function at its best. Children who eat sugary junk food at breakfast are unable to concentrate by midmorning. Kids who skip breakfast simply run out of fuel.

2. Breakfast promotes better behavior. The biggest challenge faced by many schoolchildren is not math or reading. It's controlling their behavior. It's hard to sit still and pay attention if you're hungry and your blood sugar is dropping rapidly. When blood sugar levels go up and down, so does a child's behavior, especially after going without food all night.

3. Breakfast helps keep children lean. Research has shown that children who skip breakfast or eat a junk-food breakfast are more likely to be overfat. This is because breakfast sets the nutritional tone of the day. When you begin the day with a healthy breakfast, the body is primed to stay on track for the rest of the day. Studies have confirmed that children who eat a nutritious breakfast are more likely to eat healthier food throughout the rest of the day. In contrast, children who skip breakfast or begin the day with a junk-food breakfast may compensate for the lack of good nutrition in the morning by overeating the rest of the day. Also, they are more likely to overdose on junk food, since their low blood sugar levels may set off a craving for junk carbs. Eating more calories early in the day — a nutritional concept called front-loading — seems to curb evening binges.

Studies show that people who eat a healthy breakfast eat an average of 150 fewer calories over the course of the day. It seems that calories consumed early in the day are used more efficiently, so you don't need to eat as much later. High-fiber breakfasts are especially good at helping kids stay lean. (For tips on getting kids to eat more fiber, see page 161.)

SCIENCE SAYS: BREAKFASTS BUILD SMARTER STUDENTS.

Many studies have compared children who skip breakfast, or eat junk-food breakfasts, with children who eat a healthy, balanced meal in the morning. The breakfast eaters:

- made higher grades
- were more attentive and participated better in class
- were less likely to be diagnosed with A.D.D. or learning disabilities
- had better reading and math scores
- handled complex tasks better
- missed fewer school days because of illness
- suffered less anxiety, depression, and hyperactivity
- showed improved memory

Ingredients of a Brainy Breakfast

The main ingredients of a brainy breakfast are:

- protein, which perks up the brain
- fiber-filled carbs, which provide a steady supply of fuel
- omega-3 fats, which build smart brain cells
- minerals such as calcium and iron, which help brain biochemistry work better

1. Pack in the protein. As you learned in chapter 5, protein perks up the brain by stimulating the release of the "alertness" neurotransmitters dopamine and norepinephrine. This is especially true of protein that contains the amino acid tyrosine, a neurostimulant. Protein rich in the amino acid tryptophan stimulates the release of serotonin — the calming neurotransmitter. These two T's — tyrosine and tryptophan — create balance in the brain: It's alert but also calm. The breakfast suggestions listed below include tyrosine-rich protein to wake up your child's brain in the morning. Protein is important at breakfast because of the fill-up factor, too. A high-protein breakfast keeps children from getting hungry as quickly as they do after a high-carb breakfast.

2. Get up and go with healthy carbs. Healthy carbs, such as those in fiber-filled cereals, are like time-release packets of energy. They give the brain a steady supply of fuel that keeps it humming all morning long. Junk carbs, the kind found in sugary cereals, breakfast pastries, or maple-flavored syrup, send blood sugar levels on a roller-coaster ride that causes a child's attention to wander and behavior to deteriorate. In a brainy breakfast, carbs are always partnered with protein and fiber, so the energy from the carbs is released into the bloodstream at a steady rate. The carbs we have chosen for our breakfast list below are packaged this way. For example, whole-grain waffles topped with bluberries are a brainier breakfast selection than pancakes made from white flour and topped with syrup. Here are some of our favorites:

- whole-grain waffles or pancakes topped with blueberries and peanut butter
- oatmeal with blueberries and yogurt
- whole wheat banana-nut bread and yogurt
- ½ cup low-fat cottage cheese in a scooped-out cantaloupe half
- whole-wheat tortilla wrapped around scrambled eggs and diced tomatoes
- veggie omelet, whole wheat toast, and fruit

- peanut butter and banana slices on a whole wheat English muffin with low-fat milk
- almond-strawberry yogurt cup. Layer the yogurt and strawberries (or another fruit such as blueberries or chopped apple, peaches, or pineapple) in a small bowl. Drizzle honey over the top if plain yogurt is used. Sprinkle with almonds and/or flaxseed meal.
- zucchini pancakes. This is a long-standing Sears favorite that even our toddlers enjoyed. Add a cup of shredded zucchini to whole wheat pancakes.
- smoothie (See Dr. Bill's School-Ade Smoothie, page 298.)

My nine-year-old son is very smart, but the teacher told me he gets distracted easily and doesn't pay attention like he should. I decided to try Dr. Bill's School-Ade Smoothie. I told his teacher I was going to try something different in his diet and to please let me know if there were any changes. Two weeks later the teacher called me, telling me that Louis was much more awake, was participating more in class, and was more focused. His memory and learning skills have improved. He is getting better grades on exams, and his teacher is very happy. I am, too.

MAKE BREAKFAST A HAPPY MEAL!

Help your children begin the day in a happy mood. Go to bed earlier and wake up earlier, so you are not so rushed. Stress in the morning plays havoc with brain chemistry. High levels of the stress hormone cortisol turn on the production of the neurohormone NPY, which stimulates a craving for carbs. Stress in the morning can set your child up for unhealthy eating all day long. Happy meals (no, not the fast-food type) lead to happy hormones and healthy children.

What about instant cereals? An interesting study at Children's Hospital Medical Center of Boston compared the blood sugar of children eating instant oatmeal with those eating regular oatmeal. (The oatmeals were sweetened with the same number of sugar calories.) Children served regular oatmeal had a slower rate of rise and fall in their blood sugar and felt more satisfied throughout the day. In contrast, children who ate instant oatmeal had more rapid changes in their blood sugar and ate higher-calorie snacks during the rest of the day. Avoid instant oatmeal, because the starch goes "instantly" into the bloodstream. With steel-cut, regular oatmeal, the carbs enter the bloodstream at a steadier rate.

8

Feed Your Family Immunity-Boosting Foods

Healthy foods are also healing foods. In this chapter you will learn about health foods. When we say "health foods," we don't mean the unfamiliar concoctions you might find in the aisles of your local health food store. We mean ordinary foods that research shows prevent illness and help you stay healthy. What you feed your kids can actually make a difference in how often and how severely they get sick. Parents of frequently ill children in our practice often volunteer, "You know, after eating a lot of those immune-boosting foods you recommend, he's not sick as often." Here's how to choose foods for your family that help the immune system work at peak efficiency.

FEED YOUR FAMILY LOTS OF PHYTOS

Did your grandmother frequently remind you to eat your fruits and vegetables? People have known for a long time that plant foods keep you healthy, and nutrition science is learning more and more about why. The main reason is that they contain substances called phytonutrients. *Phyton* is the Greek word for plant, and phytonutrients — phytos, for short — are immune-boosting substances found only in fruits and vegetables. Phytos are what give fruits and vegetables their rich color. Specific phytos make carrots orange, tomatoes red, blueberries blue, and spinach green. Kids like the term "phytos," as in "fighting" germs. We sometimes call them "phytomins."

When nutrition-minded moms and dads plan menus for their families, they consider the colors of the foods as well as the flavors. An entrée that includes a mixture of red, yellow, and green sweet peppers alongside orange carrots is attractive and appetizing on the plate. It's also very healthy because of the variety of phytos found in those colorful vegetables. Phytos help your body fight germs. (Tell your kids about "Phyto-Man"!) They also prevent wear and tear on your cells and organs and help the body repair itself. Unlike prescription medicines, phytos have no side effects. They do nothing but good things for you.

Teach your family about phytos. Become Phyto-Mom and Phyto-Dad. Your kids will be more excited about eating fruits and vegetables if they know why these colorful foods are so good for them. One of the goals of this book is to help children learn to appreciate the marvelous inner workings of their bodies. So teach your children about the many ways phytos help them stay healthy. Here's one way to explain to your kids the benefits of eating foods with phytos:

"Germs are like tiny

NUTSHELL

Consider fruits and vegetables your own *farm*acy.

bugs that are so small you can't even see them. Germs are what make you sick. They get inside your body and cause colds and earaches and many other kinds of sickness — even tooth decay! You can do things to keep germs out of your body. You wash your hands before eating and after going to the bathroom. You stay away from kids with colds (and if you have a cold, you cover your mouth and nose when you sneeze or cough to keep from spreading germs to your friends). Yet, no matter how careful you are to keep germs out of your body, some are going to get in. So it's important to have a strong army inside you to fight these germs.

"The germ-fighting army inside you is called your immune system. The soldiers in this army can actually chase down germs and gobble them up. If your army is strong, it will catch the germs and beat them up, but if it is tired and weak, the germs might win — and in that case, you will get sick. Your immune system army needs the good stuff in fruits, veggies, and other healthy foods to stay strong. Think of fruits and veggies as 'army food.' The better you feed your army, the better it can fight.

"These good things in fruits and vegetables called phytos help your army in other ways, too. They are like the mechanics and garbage collectors that keep the army's camp and its equipment clean and in good working order. When you get a cut or a bruise, the phytos in your army rush to the spot and get to work to help it heal. Phytos called antioxidants clean up after the army. They scrub the rust off the equipment and carry away the waste products. Other phytos are like technicians who know how to keep complicated equipment running smoothly. These phytos help your brain to think better, your eyes to see better, and your heart to pump better. They keep your skin healthy, and they help you grow."

NUTSHELL
The phytos in foods help your children muster up their own internal medicine.

We hope information about phytos motivates your family to eat more fruits and vegetables. Here are our top phyto-food picks.

TOP PHYTO FOODS

Apples
Apricots
Bell peppers (green, red, yellow)
Blueberries
Bok choy
Broccoli
Brussels sprouts
Cabbage (red, purple)
Carrots
Cauliflower
Chard
Chili peppers
Eggplant
Flaxseeds
Garlic
Grapefruit (pink)
Grapes (red, purple)
Green tea
Guava
Kale

Legumes (beans, peas, lentils)
Mangoes
Melons
Nuts
Olive oil
Onions
Oranges
Papayas
Peas (green, snow)
Pomegranates
Prunes
Radishes
Spices (e.g., turmeric, cinnamon)
Spinach or other greens
Squash
Strawberries
Sweet potatoes
Tomatoes
Vinegar

Eat a variety of phytos. Different foods contain different phytos, which have different functions in the body. For example, the beta carotene and lutein in spinach help keep eyes and skin healthy. The phytos in broccoli (e.g., vitamin C and sulforaphanes) are antioxidants; they protect rapidly growing cells from becoming

---

PILLS AND SKILLS – A NEW MEDICAL MODEL

Many people visit the doctor expecting to leave with a prescription. They believe that the best way to make themselves feel better is to take a pill. This is increasingly true for kids as well as adults. Children take pills to perk them up, pills to calm them down, pills to bring down fevers, pills for earaches, colds, and stuffy noses. Some kids and adults take pills they don't even need. Many adults prefer to take a pill to lower their cholesterol rather than to make changes in their diet and lifestyle.

As pediatricians, we know that there are times when pills are necessary, but people who are trying to get healthy need skills as well. When you're sick or have a health problem, skills can help you muster up your body's own internal medicine, its own natural ways of healing. Often this means changing how you eat, think, and live. This is challenging, but it brings better, longer-lasting, and more far-reaching results. There may be times when pills are still needed, but pills alone are rarely the answer. The best medicine comes from skills or skills plus pills. We want you to teach your children that if prescription medicines are necessary, they should always be used in addition to, not instead of, self-help skills.

---

cancerous. The list is endless. Eat lots of phyto foods together in a multifruit smoothie (see Dr. Bill's School-Ade recipe, page 298) or a salad with lots of veggies (see Dr. Bill's Super Salad recipe, page 308). When you put a bunch of phytos together you create *synergy:* all the phytos work together, so the whole is greater than the sum of its parts.

Eat phytos as close to their natural form as possible. Usually raw fruits and vegetables have more phytos than cooked vegetables,

This pills-and-skills approach puts the doctor in the role of teacher, which is what the word "doctor" originally meant in Latin. We use the pills-and-skills model in our pediatric practice, especially with children who have chronic illnesses such as asthma and diabetes or a learning problem such as A.D.D. It's important for these kids to learn that they have some control over their illness or problem. Over time, parents and children come to rely less on pills and more on their own skills. In fact, we sometimes refuse to refill a prescription for the pills unless the patient also practices the skills, especially improving their nutrition.

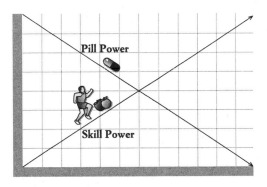

and certainly more than processed ones. But in the case of tomatoes, cooking actually helps release more phytos, such as lycopene. Lightly steaming vegetables preserves more of their nutrients. Boiling them in lots of water for a long time can destroy many of their nutrients.

Choose deep colors and strong flavors. In general, the deeper the color and the stronger the flavor, the greater the health benefits of the phyto. Tomatoes, red grapes, blueberries, Brussels sprouts, chili peppers, garlic, onions, and curry are all good sources of phytos.

FEED YOUR FAMILY FISH AND FLAX

In our medical practice we often quip, "If kids ate more fish, more doctors could go fishing." Fish and flaxseed, those top-rated fats from chapter 4, are good for your immune system as well as your nervous system. Omega-3 fats, especially those found in fatty cold-water fish, boost the immune system by helping white cells gobble up bacteria. The nutrients in fish and flaxseed help injured tissues repair themselves and fight against inflammation, which may be their most important job. You will read more about inflammation later in this chapter.

KEEP YOUR FAMILY FREE OF EXCESS INFLAMMATION

Inflammation is the current buzzword in the health field. New insights into the way many chronic diseases start reveal that inflammation is both good and bad. Of course, it protects and heals the body, but prolonged or excessive inflammation can cause excessive wear and tear on tissues, leading eventually to serious health problems. Controlling inflammation is now the focus for treating and preventing certain diseases. Taking pills is one way to control inflammation, but you can also learn skills to protect your family from excess inflammation. What you eat and how you live can protect your body from the bad kind of inflammation.

Understanding the inflammatory response. Suppose you cut your finger. At the site of the injury, local cells send out chemical messengers such as cytokines and histamines, which prompt the inflammatory response. The immune system sends an army of infection fighters to the place where the skin is broken and germs threaten to invade the body.

At the site of the invasion, local cells called macrophages ("big eaters") engulf the germs, swallowing them up to keep them from entering the body. Redness and swelling in the area result, caused by the extra capillary blood flowing to the injury site. All this commotion generates a lot of heat, so the injured area feels hot. In fact, the word *inflammation* means "a fire within." Having an inflammatory disease is like having tiny fires burning throughout the body. What does fire do? It can "burn up" germs, but it can also damage healthy tissues.

Sometimes, for reasons yet unknown, the body overreacts and sends a big army to fight a little infection, or it attacks something that isn't really a threat, such as pollen or mold. The symptoms you experience when this happens are not the fault of the germ or allergen. Instead they're caused by an overzealous immune system's inflammatory response. Sometimes the body's immune system gets confused and attacks its own tissues. The chemicals released by the inflammatory response end up damaging cells, and debris may build up in the blood vessels, leading to heart attacks or strokes, or in the brain, causing Alzheimer's disease or other neurological problems. Because of the constant work they have to do, tissues that line important highways and intersections of the body

 NUTSHELL
One of the most valuable "preventive medicine" concepts is helping your children develop a balanced immune system.

are especially vulnerable to inflammation. Joints (arthritis), intestines (colitis), breathing passages (bronchitis or asthma), and blood vessels (atherosclerosis) get "rough edges" when they are chronically inflamed, and the result can be pain and disease. The key to a healthy immune response is balance. You want your immune system to do a good job fighting infections and repairing the normal wear and tear on tissues, but you don't want it to trigger inflammation that damages healthy tissues.

Seven Ways to Keep the Body in Inflammatory Balance

Once upon a time inflammatory diseases were mostly limited to older persons. We pediatricians are seeing more of these "-itis" illnesses in kids. For example, in children, the incidence of asthma–now known to be primarily an inflammatory problem — has doubled in the past twenty years. Eczema, an inflammatory skin condition, is more common than ever. This trend is alarming yet preventable.

Inflammation is the cause of blood vessel disease, joint problems, and neurological problems that crop up more commonly as people get older. When the inflammatory response is out of whack in kids, it's an indication that their bodies are aging much too quickly. You want to send your children into adulthood with healthy blood vessels, joints, brains, and intestines, and breathing passages that work well. Fortunately, diet and lifestyle can make a big difference. Here are seven ways to help your family keep inflammation in balance.

1. Reduce your waist. Stay lean. You may think of excess fat as globs of extra tissue that just sit around on your child's waist but do nothing harmful. In fact, these fat cells are chemical factories, pumping out pro-inflammatory substances (into the bloodstream) like undisciplined soldiers in an overstaffed, restless army who go around picking fights with whoever crosses their path. The body, in its wisdom, recognizes these excess fat cells as detrimental to its health and therefore tries to fight them. The result is inflammation. The fewer the fat cells, the less inflammation. It's as simple as that. Studies have shown that the higher a person's excess body fat, the higher the risk of inflammation.

Excess internal abdominal fat is especially potent as a source of pro-inflammatory chemicals. Fat stored inside the abdomen is called visceral fat, and it spews out even more of the chemicals that promote inflammation all over the body.

Young people who want to delay getting older and old people wanting to enjoy healthy aging should keep from getting overfat to cut down on wear and tear in their tissues. In a nutshell, the fatter you are, the sooner you wear out. (See the related section Toxic Waist, page 222.)

2. Change your oils. Omega-3 oils, especially those found in cold-water fish such as salmon, trout, and herring, are the most effective anti-inflammatory foods you can eat. These healthy oils protect all tissues of the body from damage, especially the blood vessels. Just as a well-traveled road gets bumpy, the inside of your arteries gets rough. Instead of being smooth like Teflon, the arterial lining becomes more like Velcro; and like Velcro, the lining collects debris — in this case, fatty deposits called plaque. The body sends out its repair crew to smooth over the roughness. This is the body's inflammatory response. Sometimes the repair crew overdoes it, and the patch makes a big bump on the wall of the artery that can obstruct blood flow and put a person at risk for a heart attack or stroke. Omega-3 fats act like anti-inflammatories and anticoagulants to help keep the arterial lining smooth and the blood flowing. Aspirin and prescription drugs can also do this, but they can cause side effects. Remember, one of the goals of this book is to help growing bodies muster up their own preventive medicines.

Unlike fish oils and most plant oils, which are anti-inflammatory, an excess of some oils is pro-inflammatory. To keep your body in optimal health, you need to have the right balance of anti-inflammatory oils (omega 3's, like DHA and EPA) and pro-inflammatory oils (omega 6's, like arachidonic acid, or

AA), in as close to a 1:1 ratio as possible. Yet the standard American diet is a very pro-inflammatory diet. Instead of a 1:1 ratio, or even a 4:1 ratio, the ratio of pro-inflammatory to anti-inflammatory oils in the SAD diet can become 20:1 or even greater! (For more about these oils, see chapter 4.)

The best anti-inflammatory oils are the omega-3 fatty acids, specifically DHA (docosahexaenoic acid) and EPA (eicosapentaenoic acid), which are found in seafood, especially cold-water fish such as wild salmon, trout, and herring, and in seaweed (kelp, nori). Pro-inflammatory fatty acids include those in animal fat and certain plant-based oils. The most unhealthy oils are the partially hydrogenated oils, also known as trans fatty acids. Besides being pro-inflammatory, trans fats can interfere with the anti-inflammatory actions of the healthy fats such as omega 3's. See Healing Foods vs. Inflammatory Foods, opposite, to know who the bad guys are.

3. Feed your family healing instead of hurting foods. Healing foods are the grow foods you learned about in chapter 5. They contain nutrients that promote the growth of healthy tissues, strengthen the immune system to fight germs, and repair worn-out or damaged tissues. Hurting foods retard optimal growth, weaken the immune system, and promote tissue damage rather than repair.

4. Stabilize your insulin. As you learned in chapters 3 and 6, the two best ways to keep insulin levels stable are to eat healthy carbs and to graze on frequent mini-meals rather than gorge on big meals. Junk carbs tend to promote inflammation. They cause high insulin levels, which trigger the release of some of the body's most powerful pro-inflammatory substances. Insulin also promotes the storage of excess calories as fat, and excess fat (especially the flab around the waist inside the abdomen) churns out

HEALING FOODS VS. INFLAMMATORY FOODS

Some foods heal, some foods in excess can hurt.

Anti-inflammatory Foods
(Foods that promote inflammatory balance)

Pro-inflammatory Foods
(Foods that promote inflammatory imbalance)

Anti-inflammatory Foods	Pro-inflammatory Foods
Chili peppers	Animal fats in meat and dairy products, especially non-free-range animals
Cold-water fish, especially wild salmon, trout, herring	
Fish oil	Corn oil †
Flaxseeds, ground	Partially hydrogenated oils
Flaxseed oil	Safflower oil †
Fruits	Soybean oil †
Olive oil *	Sunflower oil †
Nuts *	Trans fats
Sesame oil	Foods made with the above oils, including commercial salad dressings, french fries, fast foods, most margarines, and shortening
Spices, e.g., turmeric, cinnamon, ginger	
Vegetables	
Whole grains	
Wild game meats, e.g., venison	High-fructose corn syrup

Labeling individual foods as pro- or anti-inflammatory oversimplifies the issue. The effects of a food on inflammation depend on many factors, including the foods eaten with it.

* Monounsaturated fats such as those found in nuts, avocados, and olive oil are known as neutral inflammatories, meaning they are unlikely to directly throw the inflammatory response out of balance. Yet, by putting more of these healthy fats in your diet, you are more likely to eat less of the pro-inflammatory fats, so that even monounsaturated fats can indirectly benefit your body's inflammatory response.
† While the original food and seed sources of these oils are healthy, the processing, such as hydrogenation, can render the resulting oils pro-inflammatory.

DON'T BE AN iBOD

iBod: a person who is full of inflammation or "-itis," known by the following characteristics:

- tends to be overfat (see page 211 for other medical problems)
- tends to have a big waist size, carrying extra weight around the middle
- eats lots of junk food
- overeats: eats several large meals a day instead of frequent mini-meals
- eats a lot more meat than fish
- eats more packaged foods than fresh foods
- eats at fast-food restaurants frequently
- eats insufficient fruits and vegetables
- drinks sweetened beverages instead of water

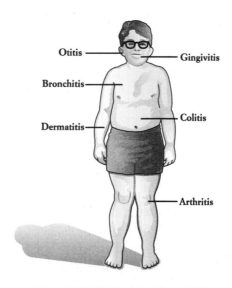

more pro-inflammatory chemicals. Studies show that people who eat a diet high in processed carbohydrates, especially those who are prediabetic or show a blood chemistry profile of insulin resistance, tend to have higher levels of inflammatory chemicals in their bloodstream. We call them iBods.

5. Move! Exercise regulates the inflammatory response in several ways:

- *Exercise stabilizes insulin.* Building more muscle tissue helps you burn more carbs, which keeps blood insulin levels lower.

- *Exercise burns fat.* The leaner you are, the lower the levels of pro-inflammatory chemicals in your blood.

- *Exercise stimulates the body to produce its own anti-inflammatory medicines,* like prostaglandins and nitric oxide, or NO (see page 187). Exercise blocks the enzyme that converts vegetable oils such as corn, safflower, and sunflower into potent pro-inflammatory substances.

6. Spice up your child's eating. You can spice up your family's health by spicing up your diet. Herbs and spices such as turmeric, ginger, cilantro, oregano, rosemary, and thyme, and pungent foods such as onions, garlic, and chili peppers have significant anti-inflammatory and antioxidant properties. Researchers studying turmeric and curry powder (a mixture of spices that includes turmeric) have found that these spices are anti- just about everything you don't want to see happen in your child's body. They improve circulation by keeping blood platelets from sticking together. They protect the liver from toxic substances. They have anti-inflammatory and antioxidant properties that help to keep all the tissues of the body healthy, including the lining of the intestines and blood vessels.

During my (Dr. Bill's) recovery from cancer surgery, I did a lot of reading about what to eat to prevent a recurrence. Turmeric was the most-mentioned spice in the medical literature I read. Turmeric seems to act like a natural version of a newer group of anti-inflammatory drugs (some of which have been taken off the market) but without the side effects!

How do you get children to accept these strong flavors? Start gradually, adding herbs and spices to familiar favorites such as casseroles and pizza. You want to shape your children's tastes toward liking spicy food. You'll give them the gift of health and also nurture a sense of adventure about eating.

7. Stay calm. New insights into the connection between mental and physical health definitely show that the nervous system and the immune system interact with each other. Excessive and unresolved stress raises the levels of stress hormones, in particular cortisol, in the bloodstream. Too much cortisol circulating in the bloodstream for too long tilts the body into a pro-inflammatory state — that is, hurting rather than healing. There are many ways to relieve stress so that your body stays relaxed and healthy. Try exercise, meditation, or perhaps just goofing around together as a family. (For family relaxation tips, see www.AskDrSears.com/relaxationtips.)

Some families need professional help to keep the relationship dynamics among family members healthy. All the healthy eating, exercise, and lifestyle changes you make can be undone if stress from difficult attitudes is allowed to get out of control. One example of this is what happens in a family when divorce or substance abuse occurs. Behavior problems also can be more than simple learning problems. If you think this could be happening in your family, because you observe depression or anxiety in yourself or your child, don't put off finding a qualified counselor or therapist who can work with you to restore the balance your family deserves.

*   *   *

In this chapter we have given you the tools to plant a doctor inside your growing child and to help each family member muster up his or her own internal medicine. In the next chapter, you will learn about another health tool — leanness.

9

Raise a Lean Family

One of the most important things you and your family can do to stay healthy is to make a commitment to staying lean. When we say "lean," we don't mean thin or skinny. By lean we mean having the right amount of body fat for your body type. Some people (kids included) must make a greater effort than others to stay lean, but it's worth it. A lean child is likely to enjoy a longer and healthier life.

HOW BIG IS THE OBESITY EPIDEMIC?

The surgeon general of the United States has described obesity as the number-one childhood health problem. The U.S. Centers for Disease Control (CDC) have stated that "childhood obesity is more serious than any infectious disease epidemic we have ever faced." The CDC warns that one in three children born in the year 2000 will become diabetic at some point in their lives if American families don't make changes in their diet and lifestyle.

During the past thirty years the number of American children who are overweight has tripled. Currently up to 25 percent of American children are overweight. In the past ten years the number of children who are overweight has jumped by over 50 percent among whites, and by more than 120 percent among Hispanics and African Americans. Here's why public health officials are so concerned:

- Children who are overweight at age eight have a 25 percent chance of becoming overweight adults.

- Eighty percent of obese adolescents remain obese throughout their lives.

- Obesity-related diseases are the leading cause of death in America.

- According to a 1999 study, 60 percent of overweight five- to ten-year-olds were found to have early signs of cardiovascular disease.

- In the past decade, hospitalizations of children for obesity-related illnesses have more than tripled.

Obesity now has its own insurance code, making it officially a disease in the eyes of the health-care industry. Parents, this is what the SAD (standard American diet) is doing to our children. The good news is that even though childhood obesity is now the number-one disease in our country, it is also the most preventable one.

HOW BEING OVERFAT CAN MAKE KIDS OVERSICK

The medical definitions of the terms "overweight" and "obese" are based on a person's weight in relation to height. We prefer to use the term "overfat" in this book, because it focuses attention on what's happening inside a child's body rather than on numbers, size, or appearance.

Whenever we talk to a group of parents, we ask them to name all the diseases they immunize their children against. Of course they mention the usual ones, such as polio, diphtheria, measles, tetanus, and chicken pox. We say, "You're missing one!" Finally we get to the point: "Immunizing your children against the modern epidemics of diabetes, heart disease, behavioral problems, learning disabilities, cancer, and mood disorders means helping them stay lean." In this chapter you will learn how to "immunize" your children against what is now the number-one childhood disease — obesity. An overfat child grows up physically, emotionally, and intellectually disadvantaged. From head to toe, here's why being overfat can lead to being underhealthy:

It bothers growing brains and emotions. Obese children suffer more headaches, learning disabilities, and emotional problems than children of normal weight. They also tend to have poorer self-images, perhaps because they are less accepted by their peers. In one study, kids were shown pictures of children with such various disabilities as missing limbs, facial and other bodily deformities, and being confined to a wheelchair. They were also shown pictures of children who were obese. When asked which

NUTSHELL
Focus on Fitness
In our LEAN Kids Program, the weight-management program at our pediatric practice, we have learned a very important weight-management tip for children: Don't emphasize scale weight or appearance. Instead, focus on fitness and performance. We first determine what the child's interest is (e.g., to run faster). We then refer to his "Run Faster Program."

of these kids they would least want to play with, they listed the "fat kids" as the least desirable playmates. Overfat kids may feel left out at school socially and on sports teams. In the media, "thin is in," which makes it hard for kids who are not thin to see themselves in a positive light and hard for their lean peers to appreciate them as individuals. As a result, obese children tend to have a poor sense of self-worth, and they wind up sitting more, eating more, and gaining more fat.

It weakens little eyes. The same nutritional excesses and deficiencies that bother the brain can also weaken the eyes. Many children who are overfat need to wear glasses because they tend to have weaker eyesight, termed "nutritional amblyopia." This is understandable, since the retina of the eye is part of the brain.

It harms growing hearts. As we have said, excess abdominal fat spews out chemicals that damage blood vessels. In addition, lugging around extra fat strains the heart. It has to work harder to pump blood around a bigger body. The heart of an overfat child works hard even when the body is at rest, causing the child to be in a constant state of "heart overload." When it needs to put forth extra effort during intense exercise, the heart may not be able to rise to the challenge. The child is exhausted long before the soccer game is over. He feels like a failure, and he may even have to endure the taunts of unkind teammates. As a result, he stops playing soccer and misses out on the exercise.

The inability of obese children to run around and play for very long may be due to damaging changes that are going on in the blood vessels that nourish the heart muscles. In fact, recent studies show that the heart's ability to pump blood to the body (called left ventricular function) tends to be weaker in obese children.

In addition, excess body fat leads to excess fat in the bloodstream. Specifically, three changes occur that are known to be associated with an increased risk of coronary artery disease:

- Total triglycerides (the total fats in the bloodstream) increase.
- Levels of LDL (the bad cholesterol that clogs arteries) go up.
- Levels of HDL (the good cholesterol that cleans arteries) go down.

A landmark study of fourteen thousand children ages five to seventeen, called the Bogalusa Heart Study, revealed that 48 percent of obese children already had one or more risk factors for cardiovascular disease, including high cholesterol, high triglyceride levels, and high blood pressure. Autopsy studies of children dying in accidents showed fatty deposits in the coronary arteries in

NUTSHELL
SAD Causes CAD
The standard American diet leads to coronary artery disease.

some children as young as one year of age. Another study showed the presence of fatty streaks in the aortas of 29 percent of children under one year of age. In children between one and nine years, fatty streaks were found in the coronary arteries of 3 percent. With these fatty deposits comes an eventual increased risk of heart attack and stroke.

It makes little lungs tired. Lugging around extra body fat makes it harder to breathe. Overfat kids find it takes more effort to inhale. This is called the obesity-hypoventilation syndrome. Children don't take in as much air with each breath as they should, so they get winded easily, especially during sports. Since obesity also depresses immunity, obese children are more prone to respiratory illnesses such as colds, bronchitis, and asthma.

MORE FAT, LESS SLEEP

Excess fat that accumulates in the tissues around the breathing passages can partially obstruct the airways, making it harder to breathe. Fat bothers breathing more at night because the airways automatically relax and become more narrow during sleep. This breathing difficulty is called sleep apnea. A child with this condition breathes noisily and irregularly during sleep, with occasional long pauses of fifteen to twenty seconds between breaths (which seems like an eternity to someone listening). Then the child wakes up partially and takes a loud catch-up breath. These waking-to-breathe episodes lead to restless sleep and tired brains and bodies the next day.

Sleep apnea can be treated in a number of ways. Weight loss helps. Talk to your doctor if you suspect that your child has sleep apnea. A video of your child sleeping may help you show the doctor what you're concerned about.

It tricks little tummies. Excess fat inside the abdomen puts extra pressure on a full stomach. That's why overfat children and adults tend to have more problems with gastroesophageal reflux disease (GERD), most often described as heartburn, when the pressure in the abdominal cavity causes stomach acids to back up into the esophagus. For overfat people, eating is associated with feelings of discomfort, indigestion (especially when they are lying down), and painful night waking.

It bothers growing bones. During checkups, overfat children often tell us things like this: "I waddle when I walk, and I don't like it." "My knees and hips hurt when I run." "My feet are always sore at the end of gym class." Extra weight can stress bones and joints, so many overfat children develop bowed legs or turned-in knees. The excess weight makes their feet sore. They have flat feet and endure pain on the bottom of their heel bones. For this reason, we advise parents to put heel cushions in the shoes of overfat children. These kids may need to wear orthotics or arch supports to keep their feet from turning in, which throws their knees out of alignment. These precautions are especially important in children who do a lot of running on hard surfaces, such as asphalt or gym floors made of tile laid on cement. Being overfat also puts kids at an increased risk of injury. One of the most painful sports injuries I (Dr. Bill) ever attended as a team doctor was a dislocated hip in an overfat tackle on a high school football team. This student athlete's size put him at risk for this terribly painful injury.

It damages young hormones, causing diabetes. Insulin-resistant diabetes, once seen almost exclusively in adults, is appearing in kids at younger ages. Obesity puts them at risk. Excess fat cells in the body produce substances that contribute to the development of insulin resistance. When cells resist insulin, blood sugar levels rise and the pancreas cranks out more and more insulin to force the sugar from the blood into the cells. Insulin levels tend to be higher in people with a higher body mass index, or BMI (a measure of obesity calculated from height and weight). Eventually, the pancreas wears out, and the person has to get shots of insulin to control blood sugar levels.

The new term for obesity-triggered diabetes is "diabesity," which reinforces the strong link between obesity and the development of insulin-resistant diabetes. Because of this association, pediatricians are starting to consider every child who is overfat, especially those with excess weight around their middles, as being pre-diabetic. While this term may be scary, it's scary for a reason. It's a reminder that overfat children need to change the way they eat and live if they want to avoid full-blown diabetes.

It gets young bodies off track. Besides being prone to major medical problems associated with obesity, overfat children tend to suffer a variety of other medical nuisances. They may have dry, flaky, bumpy skin. They may get infections or experience chafing in the folds of excess fat, especially in the buttocks, groin, and neck. They are at higher risk for gallbladder disease. Overfat children also have more problems during puberty, because excess fat affects the levels of sex hormones. Overweight girls tend to develop earlier but have more irregular menstrual periods. They may also show masculine features such as rougher skin and coarse facial hair. Males may experience delayed puberty. In addition, they may be embarrassed by the development of large, fatty breasts and excess folds of pelvic fat that partially obscure the penis, making it look underdeveloped.

IS YOUR CHILD AT RISK FOR OBESITY? HOW TO TELL

How intensely you need to practice lean eating in your family depends upon your family's level of risk. Consider these factors:

Risky family genes. Is your family tree weighed down with obese persons? Or do you come from a long line of lean relatives? While eating habits are more important than genes (you can change habits!), heredity does play an important part in determining your body type and your tendency to store fat. If both parents are overfat, their children have an 80 percent chance of becoming overfat themselves. If one parent is overfat, the children have a 40 percent chance. If neither parent is overfat, the child has only a 7 percent chance of being overfat. The passing down of eating patterns from parent to child explains part of this tendency for weight problems to run in families, but not all of it.

Risky body types. People come in all sizes and shapes. What a boring world it would be if we didn't. Yet some of these body types are more likely to carry excess weight than others. Some body types tend to be calorie burners and others calorie storers. Those who burn calories more easily stay lean with less effort than those who tend to store calories. Body types are often compared to fruit:

- *Bananas* are people who are naturally slender and often tall, with no excess body fat, especially around the middle. They burn lots of calories without even thinking about it. Bananas tend to automatically adjust their eating habits to their calorie needs. They eat less when they are less active.

- *Apples* are people of average height and weight who tend to store excess weight around their middles. They are usually more muscular than bananas but tend to be fat storers. Apple have the highest risk of becoming obese, and the abdominal fat they accumulate places them at higher risk for heart disease and diabetes. They find it hard to cut back on food when they are less active.

- *Pears* are short and wider in the hips and thighs. Pears, like apples, tend to store calories rather than burn them and are also more likely than bananas to become overfat.

- *Yams* are just plain big from head to toe. After apples, yams are the body type most prone to becoming overfat.

Not all children and adults fit neatly into these four categories, but you can use them to determine general tendencies. For example, if both of your family trees are full of bananas, yet your eight-year-old healthy eater is pleasingly plump, you probably don't need to worry. Many children go through a "chunky" stage from seven to ten years of age. They are storing up energy for the

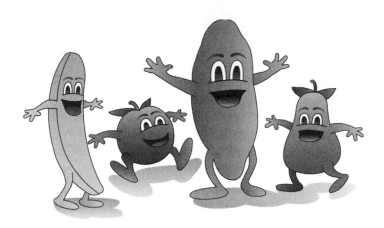

growth spurts of the preteen and teenage years, when they eventually "lean out."

We recently saw two children in our practice from the same family. Despite similar diets, one of the girls is a lean "banana" and the other is an "apple." "No fair," said Susan, the apple. "My sister gobbles banana splits, yet I'm a size sixteen and she's a size eight." One girl got the calorie-burning genes; the other got the calorie-storing ones.

Risky family eating habits. Which aisles do you frequent in the supermarket? Do you spend your shopping time selecting produce, or do you linger in the aisles with all the prepackaged crackers and cookies? Do you plan to have healthy family meals at home, or does the dinner hour find you in the drive-up lane at a fast-food outlet? Do a lot of the foods in your pantry or refrigerator have one or more of the three "bad words" ("high-fructose corn syrup," "hydrogenated," or a color additive, like red #40) on the label? Is health and nutrition a high or low priority in your family? Finally, do the parents in your family (you!) eat the way you want your kids to eat? Monkey see, monkey do. Little monkeys learn their eating habits from the big monkeys.

HELPING CHILDREN LIKE THEIR BODIES

The glamorously thin performers and models on television, in the movies, and in magazines present culturally idealized body types that leave today's kids, especially teens and preteens, unhappy with their own bodies. It's important for kids to have a realistic body image, and to be comfortable with the bodies they have. Here are some rules:

- *Never tease your child about his or her body,* and don't allow kids to criticize other kids' bodies. Avoid negative words and nicknames like "Shorty," "Skinny," "Chubby," "Klutz," and so on.

- *Help your child take pride in what his or her body can do,* whether it's being a good soccer player, a good dancer, or someone who takes long hikes on a family vacation. You don't have to be a great athlete to enjoy being healthy and strong. Tell your child, "I love to see you run" or "It's fun to watch you dance. You seem to love what you're doing."

Your child's temperament. Lively, active children burn more calories than kids who prefer to sit and play video games. Some children are naturally wiggly. Others like to sit still. Obviously, a child who prefers to read books and do art projects will burn fewer calories than a child who spends hours chasing a soccer ball or a sibling around the backyard. Parents may have to get quieter children involved in activities that encourage them to be more active.

Doctor's evaluation. If you're concerned that your child is over-fat or at risk for becoming so, talk to your doctor. The doctor will

- *Help your child look at the situation realistically.* Kids are sensitive about their bodies. They notice if they're shorter, taller, skinnier, or have bigger feet than most kids their age. For example, almost every preteen and teenage girl in America thinks she needs to lose weight. Most don't, and parents can remind these fat-phobic young women that their bodies are very nice just the way they are.

- *Help your child make changes.* If your child would benefit from more exercise and less junk food, help him or her to make the needed changes. Don't emphasize appearance. Instead, tell your child that eating better means better thinking, better running, better performance all around, and better feeling.

- *Find ways to turn negative feelings into positive ones:* "Dad didn't grow to be six feet tall until he was out of high school." "You are so graceful. You make that dress look really elegant." Point out that your child is creative or a good friend or a determined hardworking member of the sports team and tell him or her how important these qualities are for success in life.

assess your child's height and weight and use these numbers to determine his or her BMI (body mass index; see page 216). The doctor may also take note of your child's waist circumference. We often do a "pinch test," that is, we determine how much extra fat there is around a child's middle by seeing how much we can gently grab. We personally find this to be the most meaningful measurement, yet admittedly, it is less objective than the numbers on the scale. Your doctor will also consider age, stage of development, family history, and diet and activity level as all three of you decide together what to do about your child's weight.

TOXIC WAIST

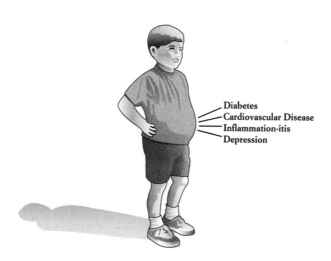

Diabetes
Cardiovascular Disease
Inflammation-itis
Depression

A "spare tire" around the middle is more than just dead weight. The more fat that shows around the waistline, the more fat is stored inside the abdomen, around vital organs. This fat is called visceral fat, and it behaves differently from fat stored elsewhere on the body. You could call this middle fat "toxic waist" because it is more metabolically active than fat in other parts of the body. What it does is release health-harming chemicals into the bloodstream, chemicals that affect your body in many ways.

Fat cells can be both good and bad. They are good guys when there are not too many of them and they are used for fuel. However, extra fat cells, especially those that reside around the waist, are like mad scientists turned loose in the laboratory that is your body. These cells are like factories, churning out bad chemicals and releasing them into your bloodstream, where they can increase your risk of heart disease, stroke, cancer, diabetes, and premature aging. Here's how:

- Fat cells release substances that are pro-inflammatory. They damage tissues, aging them prematurely — not what you want for your growing children.

- Other substances released by fat cells can cause blood clots, which block tiny blood vessels, preventing blood from flowing to vital organs that need optimal amounts of nutrients from the blood for optimal growth.

- Excess fat cells manufacture chemicals called vasoconstrictors that narrow the blood vessels and raise blood pressure. An excess of fat cells also inhibits the body's release of nitric oxide, which helps relax blood vessels. Lower nitric oxide levels contribute to high blood pressure.

- Some studies indicate that fat cells may manufacture chemicals that increase a person's risk of getting cancer. We know that fat cells increase estrogen levels in the body, and this may affect cancer risk. (High estrogen levels may also be why overfat girls experience puberty sooner than lean ones.)

- Fat cells release chemicals that make healthy cells in the body more resistant to insulin, thus greatly increasing the risk of diabetes.

Middle fat is a good news/bad news scenario. You've already read the bad news. The good news is that it's the first fat to go when you get more exercise and start eating lean. This is why in our pediatric practice we are more concerned about waist size than scale measurements. We tell children to shoot for "looser jeans" rather than a target weight on the scale.

SAD SODAS

Soda is everywhere. It's impossible to avoid the ad campaigns, the special offers, and the suggestion that it's a great snack and a suitable accompaniment to every meal. How do you get kids to understand the nutritional truth about these bad-for-you beverages? Give them the facts, and teach them to be smarter than all those junk-food ads that are trying to sell kids something they're better off without. And refuse to buy it.

Some parents are not convinced of the health hazards of sweetened beverages, especially for growing children. To make this point in our pediatric office, we recently displayed four giant-size bottles of the junkiest of sweetened beverages on our check-out counter. We printed up a label for each of the bottles that read "Diabetes in a Bottle." We then watched the shock register on parents' faces as they walked by our graphic message. They seemed to get the point.

Here are the facts to share with your kids:

- *Soda weakens your bones.* It contains a chemical called phosphate, which is what makes it fizzy. Phosphate likes to pair up with calcium, so when it gets into your body, it steals calcium from your bones.

- *One can of soda contains 10 teaspoons of sugar.* Would you ever eat this much sugar out of a sugar bowl? You'd feel yucky if you

TEN WAYS TO RAISE A LEAN CHILD

Children get overfat when they eat too much of the wrong kinds of food and don't burn off the calories. Changing what children eat and how active they are will get them lean. It's as simple as that! Here are the specifics:

did, and soda makes you feel yucky, too. If you pay attention to how you feel after you drink it, you'll see that. It's the fizzy effect that takes your mind off how yucky the sugary liquid really is.

- *Soda makes you fat.* Did you ever notice that you feel hungry — very hungry — shortly after you finish drinking a can of pop? (After you burp, that is!) You might feel like you want to eat a whole bag of potato chips. You feel this way because the soda doesn't really satisfy your hunger.

- *Soda comes in many colors* — orange, yellow-green, brown. It's not naturally any of those colors. The colors come from chemical dyes that could be bad for you.

- *Soda gives you cavities.* The acids in soda damage the enamel that protects your teeth from decay.

- *Soda is not cool.* The companies that make soda use television commercials and other kinds of advertising to make it seem like soda is the cool thing for kids to drink. They make lots of money by selling you something that is not good for you. Wouldn't you like to outsmart them by not buying their product? Do it! Really, it's cool to say no to junk drinks.

1. Feed your child lean carbs. Once upon a time, fats were the foods blamed for widening waistlines. New research implicates carbs as another culprit. Kids need carbs for energy to grow and play and learn, but some carbs help them stay lean, while others make them fat. A "lean carb" is one that comes with proteins, fiber, and/or moderate amounts of healthy fat. Lean carbs release

---

LOW FAT BUT HIGH CARB

"Low fat" on the front of the package does not necessarily translate into less fat on a child's body. Fats carry much of the flavor in food, so when manufacturers take out fat, they often add more sugar to make up for the difference in taste. So "low fat" may mean higher carbs. If the food was full of junk carbs to begin with, the low-fat version won't be any better for you than the original. Examine the Nutrition Facts box on the package. If the carb food has fewer than 2 grams of protein or fiber, chances are it's a fat carb. If the words "corn syrup" or "high-fructose corn syrup" appear on the ingredients list, you can be sure these are fat carbs. Leave the package on the shelf. After all, what good is a low-fat Twinkie?

---

energy at a steady rate, because the protein, fiber, and fat slow their digestion. These partner nutrients also make lean carbs filling. A "fat carb," on the other hand, is a high-sugar food with little or no fiber, protein, or healthy fat. Fat carbs are digested quickly and send the blood sugar on a roller-coaster ride — up to the heights and quickly down again. Hunger follows, with a craving for more fat carbs.

Lose the liquid candy. Sweetened beverages are one of the main contributors to the epidemic of childhood obesity. In fact, studies by the U.S. Department of Agriculture (USDA) suggest that high-fructose corn syrup (HFCS) not only contributes to childhood obesity but may also be generally harmful to health. HFCS is no better than liquid candy. Anything made with this fat carb is something you should definitely leave on the shelf at the supermarket, especially if you have a child who is trying to get lean.

2. Trim the food fat. The best fats for kids trying to get lean are the omega-3 fats found in seafood. Fats from plant sources are also good lean foods, but even healthy oils such as olive oil can make you fat if you overindulge. For a leaner, healthier family, limit the amount of fat, especially saturated fat, in your family's menus. (Saturated fat is the kind found in foods from animal sources.) Try these fat-trimming tactics:

- Bake or broil meat, fish, and chicken, instead of frying.

- Trim the fat from poultry and meat before you cook it. Much of the fat in chicken is right under the skin. If you remove the skin, you remove most of the fat.

- Drink low-fat or nonfat (skim) milk.

- Use low-fat cheese, low-fat cottage cheese, and plain low-fat or nonfat yogurt. Don't give your overfat child sugar-sweetened yogurt. It has too many junk carbs.

- Instead of butter, use olive oil as a dip or spread for bread, or spread bread with peanut butter, almond butter, hummus, or mashed avocado.

AVOID THE "TERRIBLE TWOS"

Check the ingredients list on packaged foods and avoid those that contain either high-fructose corn syrup or hydrogenated oils. Foods that contain either one or both of these food-factory ingredients have little nutritional value and lots of empty calories. These also contribute to obesity. Avoiding foods that contain these two chemically processed ingredients is one of the most important changes you can make to get your family on track toward healthy eating. If those words are on the label, don't buy that food.

3. Fill up with fiber. Fiber is filling without being fattening. Foods that are high in fiber take up lots of room in the stomach, so you feel full when you eat them. Yet the fiber in the food is calorie-free, since the body cannot break down fiber and use it for energy. It's hard to eat too much of a high-fiber food. High-fiber foods require lots of chewing, so they cannot be eaten quickly. They stay in the stomach longer and absorb water, so you feel full longer. When high-fiber foods are part of a meal or snack, you tend to eat less of other foods, including those that are high in fat and calories.

High-fiber foods help kids get and stay lean. If your child tends to overeat at meals, offer high-fiber foods such as an apple, veggies, or salad as a pre-meal snack. She will fill up on the high-fiber foods and be less likely to overeat at dinnertime. (See the Best Fiber Foods chart, page 162.)

4. Pack on the protein. Kids are unlikely to overeat when they are eating high-protein foods. Protein slows the absorption of carbs, so you don't get the sugar rush followed by the sugar low that you get with carbs alone. Protein leaves kids feeling full and satisfied longer, and they burn calories just digesting protein. Some protein, however, comes packaged with fat, especially saturated fat, so to help kids stay lean, concentrate on lean proteins such as the following:

- beans and other legumes
- fish, especially salmon, tuna, trout, herring, and other cold-water fish
- lean meat and poultry (most of the visible fat removed)
- nonfat and low-fat dairy products
- nuts, in palm-size servings

5. Downsize your child's servings. Are your child's eyes bigger than her stomach? Portion distortion can be a problem for

SMALL CHANGES = BIG LOSS OF FAT

It's really not hard to keep kids lean. Small changes over the course of a year can add up to a significant fat loss. Eliminate just *50 calories a day* (that's one fewer sweetened beverage every three days) and a child can lose 6 pounds in a year. Ten to fifteen minutes of running every day will burn enough calories over a year to take off 6 pounds. Small changes are not hard to make, but they can make a big difference to your child's health.

grown-ups, too. Some restaurants serve what we dub "super-bowls," enormous portions of pasta, potatoes, and meat, to convince diners that they are getting a good value. What diners are really getting is enough food to make them fat (or, if they are wise, enough food to save for another meal the next day).

The younger a child is at the onset of obesity, the more serious it is. A young obese overeater is metabolically programmed to feel that she needs to overeat. This is why it is important to allow young children to follow their own hunger cues. If you urge them to keep eating even when their tummies are telling them they are full, you interfere with healthy metabolic programming. Kids who eat too much may need some gentle reprogramming.

What are appropriate-size portions for kids? A child's tummy is about the size of her fist. So a snack should be no more than a fist-size amount of food, and a meal no more than two or three fistfuls. Here are some tips to help your children be satisfied with just the right amount of food:

- Begin by redirecting your child toward fill-up foods like raw veggies. Fill-up foods contain the two most filling nutrients: protein and fiber. They satisfy the overeater with fewer calories.

- Give children smaller plates to make small portions look larger.

- Let children serve themselves. Studies show that many children who serve themselves take less food than their parents give them.

- If your child tends to overserve himself and overeat, put the food on his plate at the kitchen counter rather than setting the food in serving bowls on the dinner table. Children are less likely to ask for more if the food is not right there in front of them. Out of sight is out of mind, and if the food is out of sight, it is less likely to end up in a child's tummy. If a child typically asks for another helping of a favorite food, be sure the first helping is small enough to warrant seconds.

- Avoid asking your children, "Would you like more?" If they are hungry enough, they'll ask. You want your children to learn to listen to their own hunger cues, not to you urging them to finish up their dinner or to have more.

- Avoid pressuring your child to clean his plate. Children should decide when to stop eating based on how their tummies feel, not on how much food is left on the plate.

6. Teach your child to eat slowly. The body and brain work together to tell you when to stop eating. When the stomach is getting full, it sends out hormones to signal the appestat in the brain, saying you've eaten enough and it's time to stop. However, this is a time-delayed message. The more slowly you eat, the better this mechanism works. It takes around thirty minutes of eating before these feel-full hormones kick in. Someone who eats quickly can eat more than enough food before the brain has a chance to say "Stop!"

It's important to teach your child to eat slowly. The body's system for controlling food intake works much better if children do not rush through meals. Slowing down the pace of eating gives

ENJOY "FREE" FOODS

Children seldom get fat from eating too much grow food. Many grow foods are free foods. An "eat-all-you-want" food is one that enjoys these three perks that naturally curb overeating:

- *It is naturally a fill-up food.* Foods that are high in fiber, protein, or other nutrients make a child satisfied with smaller portions. It's hard to overeat grow foods.

- *It tends to be chewy and take longer to eat.* Grow foods make a child feel satisfied sooner. The body uses up a lot of calories just chewing and digesting these foods, especially vegetables.

- *It tends to be high in water content and/or protein.* Foods with a high water and/or protein content such as fruits and vegetables fill and satisfy hungry tummies. They are especially good for the child who tends to overeat, since it's nearly impossible to overeat a plate of vegetables and get fat on them, unless they are served with loads of butter or rich sauce.

The best free foods for children are:

- beans and other legumes
- eggs
- fruit
- oatmeal
- salmon
- tofu
- veggies
- yogurt, plain

Children and teens especially like the free foods concept because it's a positive message. "Eat all you want, it's good for you" invokes a more upbeat response than "You can't eat that." The concepts of grow foods and free foods put a positive spin on healthy eating.

children a chance to listen to their appetite-control signals. Try these slow-down-your-eating tricks:

- *Encourage your child to take small bites.* Cut his food into small pieces. Give him a salad fork instead of a full-size dinner fork. Smaller bites take longer to eat, so the stomach has enough time to signal the brain "You're full. That's enough."

- *Make mealtime and snacks a social occasion.* Some children wolf down their food because they're impatient to get the meal over with. (They've got other things to do!) Sit down and talk with your child while she has a snack or a meal. Make family meals a relaxing, friendly time when you, your child, and everyone else at the table enjoy their food and one another.

- *Hit the pause button.* Encourage your child to put down her spoon or fork and pause from time to time while she is eating. She might want to take a drink of water or milk after every few bites, or just take a few deep breaths. Ask her open-ended questions while she's eating so that she has to stop eating to answer you. Before you serve seconds, spend ten minutes in conversation. Your child's appestat will give her the full signal, and those seconds will become tomorrow's leftovers.

- *Play "chew-chew."* To get your child to eat more slowly, tell him to chew each bite at least ten times. Play a game in which you help him count how many times he chews. Chewing makes eating more enjoyable, and it makes food easier to digest. Saliva contains digestive enzymes that begin to break food down while it is still in your mouth. Chewing also breaks up the fiber that holds food together, leaving less work for the stomach acids. Well-chewed food slides along the digestive track more easily.

- *Encourage children to pay attention to their tummies.* Many kids overeat because they miss the signals from their tummy that tell them they are full. Midway through a meal, ask your child, "Are you starting to feel full?" Let him know that it's okay to stop eating when his tummy begins to feel full. Remind your child, "You'll feel yucky if you eat too much." Bite your tongue if you feel the impulse to urge your child to clean his plate. Old patterns from childhood are hard to break.

Dr. Bob shares what works with his kids:

We never make our kids finish the food on their plates. If they don't feel like eating, we act like it's no big deal. Of course, the rule is grow foods before fun foods. They don't get dessert or their favorite side dish (like French bread with butter) unless they eat their grow food first. We put no pressure on them. We save their plate for later in case they decide they're hungry.

7. Watch out for mindless munching. Television plays a big role in childhood obesity. Consider these scary facts about snacking and screen time:

- Children who watch more TV are more likely to request and purchase foods high in sugar and fat.

- Children who watch more TV tend to have a higher percentage of fat and sugar in their diets.

- Studies show that the more TV children watch, the more likely they are to be obese and to have high cholesterol levels.

Children who are sitting around watching TV are not burning up calories playing soccer, tag, or hide-and-seek. And while watching, they tend to munch mindlessly on snacks. When tuned in to the tube, children tune out their body's signals for appetite control. Kids can wolf down a whole bag of chips without realizing it.

What's more, the foods children snack on while watching television are often the wrong kinds of foods. Television commercials relentlessly push junk food at kids, giving them the impression that all kinds of questionable snacks are good for them, when really they're not. Television commercials, and programs, too, give children the message that highly processed junk food is what cool kids eat. It's up to you to set them straight. If your child does want a snack while watching a favorite television program, give him a healthy high-fiber or high-protein snack — something from the list of grow foods on page 55, not from the supermarket's junk-food displays.

We discourage parents from putting television sets in their children's bedrooms. With the TV in the bedroom, you have little control over what your kids watch and what they eat while they're watching.

8. Get kids moving. One of the magic words in keeping kids lean is "move!" We believe the two most important contributors to the epidemic of childhood obesity are too many sweetened beverages and sitting rather than moving for entertainment.

If you have a child who loves to sit and watch TV or play computer or video games, have a house rule: TIME SITTING = TIME MOVING. Better yet, make TV time move time. Have kids exercise *while* watching the tube by jumping on a mini trampoline, jumping rope, or flexing their muscles with exercise bands. Each day require your children to spend at least the same amount of time in physical play as they do sitting in front of a screen. Even a small increase in physical activity adds up to a lot more leanness. If your child is 5 to 10 pounds overfat (which many children are), moving an extra twenty to thirty minutes a day is an easy way to get rid of that extra fat in one year's time.

9. Slow down on the fast food. Let your kids know that your family rarely eats at fast-food joints. Use "we" statements: "We just don't eat that kind of food." It's no accident that fast-food restaurants are strategically located where families travel back and forth to work and school, and also where older kids tend to hang out (i.e., near middle schools and high schools). When you're hungry and in a hurry, fast food may seem like the answer. But if your whole family is struggling with being overfat, you may have to adopt strict principles about fast-food restaurants: "We don't often go there, and when we do, we still try to eat healthy." Here are some tips on eating lean while eating out.

- *Have a salad first.* Patronize restaurants that offer a salad bar with green greens, not just iceberg lettuce (for why, see page 126). Salads are filling, and they're not fattening unless they are overloaded with dressing. Beginning the meal with a healthy salad is one of the best ways to curb overeating.

- *Order small portions.* Nobody needs all the fat in a double cheeseburger. Stay away from the super-big sandwiches and stick to the smaller-size versions. Share an order of french fries rather than buying fries for each person. Tell the restaurant to hold the "special sauce," which is probably full of bad fats. Take advantage of any effort the restaurant is making to offer healthy food, such as fruit as a side dish, carrot sticks, or salads.

- *Shun sweetened beverages.* This "liquid candy" is the worst fast food because the carbs in it rush fast into the bloodstream, unlike with the "slow foods" or good carbs that are partnered with protein and fiber to slow down the rush. Restaurants make most of their money on the junk beverages and desserts that accompany a meal. That's why soda is the main beverage offering. Ask for water, milk, or 100 percent juice instead. Use the water to dilute the juice and share it. You'll save money, too! (See Eating Healthy When Eating Out, page 280.)

10. Stay lean yourself. Parents, your kids are watching you eat! You are your child's most important teacher, and children learn best from good examples. If you are passionate yourself about

NUTSHELL
Salt Doesn't Satisfy
Salt stimulates the appetite, making you want to eat more. So if your family has a hard time curbing their overeating, go easy on salt, but jazz up the food with savory spices such as curry and turmeric or with lemon juice.

eating right and staying fit, your child will adopt your good habits. You have a great deal of influence over your child in the preschool and early elementary years. Even when your child gets to be a preteen or teenager and friends become all-important, your example is still a powerful influence on your child. Take advantage of this and teach your child about healthy living by staying lean yourself.

If your family is struggling with an overfat issue, we suggest you read our book *Dr. Sears' LEAN Kids: A Total Health Program for Children Ages 6–12* (New American Library, 2003).

10

Food Shopping with Your Kids

The supermarket is a giant nutritional classroom. In this chapter, Dr. Jim shares the eye-opening experiences he and his two children had while shopping for food. Don't miss a chance like this to teach your child how to stay on the right track!

While I was preparing to talk to a parents' group about the importance of nutrition for their kids, I decided that I would take some pictures of various healthy foods and junk foods at the grocery store to illustrate my lecture. I thought it would be fun to take my kids along on this shopping trip so they could be in the pictures and learn about how to shop for healthy food. I planned on taking two trips: one to our local supermarket and one to a natural and organic foods supermarket. Off we went — the kids, the camera, and I. My kids learned some great lessons about nutrition, and I learned a lot about how food is marketed to kids. I could not believe the difference between the two trips!

BECOMING SUPERMARKET SAVVY

My kids were excited about going shopping with Dad. This was because, as they said, "Mom never takes us to the grocery store." Diane tries to go while the kids are in school. I would soon find out why.

First (unhealthy) impressions. From the moment we entered the store, we were bombarded with advertising — "Drink this" and "Buy that"! It was overwhelming. Walking through the entrance, we had to pass under an archway formed by two large stacks of soda cases bridged with a large banner that had several *Star Wars* characters pointing to the soda and proclaiming, "May the force be with you." My seven-year-old, Jonathan, is an avid *Star Wars* fan. His eyes lit up. He looked at the soda and then at Yoda and asked me, "Hey, Dad, can we get that?" Jonathan is a child who never drinks soda and doesn't even like it, and suddenly he was asking for it just because one of his heroes was on a sign. Clever marketing, I thought. Show Yoda with a soda. A line from one of the early *Star Wars* movies came to mind: "I've got a bad feeling about this." (This is what Han Solo says as he pilots his starship toward the Death Star.)

Just past the gigantic gateway of soda, we found ourselves face-to-face with a big display of candy and cookies. Now, my kids generally are good eaters — they know the importance of fruits and vegetables and of not eating too many sweets. But face-to-face with all this temptation, they were clamoring for treats. I had to acknowledge that the grocery store and food company marketing executives know exactly how to appeal to my kids. We had not been in the store for more than a minute and Jonathan and Lea had asked me for soda, candy, and cookies three or four times!

I tried to steer them quickly toward the perimeter of the store, the outer aisles and the back, where most stores put the grow foods — healthy fruits and vegetables, meat and fish, and dairy products. The problem was that to get to the produce section we had to pass the soda aisle, the candy aisle, the cereal aisle, and the juice aisle. At each point, my kids were bombarded with signs and packaging featuring their favorite cartoon and movie characters telling them to eat junk. I was getting angry. This is a store I've been in many times over the years, but I hadn't realized how much the advertising and marketing strategies were targeted at children. When I run in with my short list on my way home from work, I don't pay much attention to Darth Vader selling junk cereal. I hurry by on my way to get the things we need, usually eggs, whole wheat bread, fruit, and whatever is on the menu for dinner. But with my kids along, it was impossible to ignore all the hype.

Picking produce. We finally made it to the produce section, and Jonathan started to whine, "Why do we have to be here? I want to go back to the *Star Wars* aisle." I asked him which aisle that was. He replied, "The one with all the *Star Wars* stuff." I said, "You mean the cereal aisle?" He said, "Yes, yes, the *Star Wars* aisle." Boy, was he sucked in big-time. It was clear to me that the food industry's main concern is making money, not bringing healthy food to American consumers. I thought to myself, Wouldn't it be great if Bugs Bunny, Darth Vader, and R2-D2 were telling my kids to eat fruits and vegetables instead of sugary cereals?

"Okay, kids, let's pick out some good fruits and vegetables, and let me get some pictures of you that I can use for my slide show." Of course, my eleven-year-old daughter, Lea, was excited about this, because she wanted to see herself up on the screen during the lecture. So she grabbed a handful of apples and proudly showed them to me while I took a picture.

The apples she grabbed were her favorite ones, Pink Lady apples. She likes these because the peel is softer than on other varieties of apples. When she was younger, she didn't like apples because of the hard peel. For years, to get her to eat an apple, we would have to peel it and cut it up — a time-consuming process when you're packing lunches in the morning. And the apple chunks would be brown by lunchtime. Besides, the red peel contains a lot of phytos and fiber that she was missing out on. But at some point, Lea tried a Pink Lady apple and proclaimed, "I like this, I can eat the peel." Diane and I looked at each other and with big smiles said, "We're going to buy a lot of Pink Lady apples." So Lea's Pink Lady apples were the first thing we put in our shopping cart.

Next we found the cantaloupe. Cantaloupe is good for you. It is very rich in beta carotene, like carrots and sweet potatoes. But here again, getting our kids to eat cantaloupe was a long process. We kept offering it to them, but they would usually take a bite and say, "I don't want it. I don't like it." But we persisted, and sure enough, this year they finally started to like cantaloupe, after Diane and I had finished countless melons all by ourselves. Now they have cantaloupe for breakfast and in their school lunches several times a week.

Lettuce lessons. We needed lettuce, so we moved on to salad greens. I told Lea, "Go pick up one of those big white balls of lettuce," referring to iceberg lettuce. We opened it up and took out a leaf and held it up to the light. I said, "What's funny about this lettuce?" She looked at it and said, "I can see through it." We tried the same thing with a head of leaf lettuce, which was a deep, dark green. I said, "What do you think about this?" And she said, "It's very dark green. It must have lots of stuff that's good for you compared with the see-through lettuce."

When I was growing up, my mom bought only romaine lettuce. I had to go to a restaurant or friend's house to get iceberg lettuce in a salad or on a hamburger. I definitely preferred it to the salads my mom made, with all the "healthy stuff" she added. When I was a kid, dark lettuce just didn't seem palatable to me, but I don't want my kids to develop the same prejudice against the good stuff. So as we looked at the two lettuces, I told my son, "The dark green one will help you run really fast." To my daughter I said, "It will give you prettier hair and sharper eyes." Then I asked them, "Which lettuce would you rather have — the fast-running lettuce or the slow-running lettuce?" My seven-year-old said, "I want the fast-running lettuce," and he promptly put it into our shopping cart.

Because I had involved the kids in the decision about which lettuce to buy, I hoped they would be more inclined to eat the good lettuce. And sure enough, that night we made a healthy salad with the dark green lettuce and some other great ingredients (more about those in our recipes section), and they liked it. Yeah! That same approach can be used with a lot of fruits and vegetables. Have your kids pick out the brightest colors they can find — the deepest reds, the darkest greens, and the brightest yellows. They can get excited about trying the dark red grapes instead of the pale green ones (fortunately you can get them both seedless). You can get excited because they're getting more nutrition.

Fabulous fruits. Jonathan and Lea picked out a nice variety of fruits and vegetables. Jonathan made sure we got lots of bananas, one of his current favorites for topping breakfast cereal. We picked out some blueberries, which are good on almost everything. Diane and I like to put blueberries and yogurt on top of the steel-cut oatmeal we cook for breakfast. (Steel-cut oatmeal has a very nice, rich taste and is a great source of fiber.) We also selected some grapefruit, which my kids like. We chose the red grapefruit because the natural red color makes it a great source of the antioxidant lycopene, which is important for growing kids. Lycopene is found mainly in tomatoes, so if your picky eater won't go near grapefruit, serve tomatoes instead. Having the kids help pick out the produce we bought made a difference when we got home. They remembered it was there, and they ate it.

YUMMY YOGURT

What food processors have done to yogurt is a shame. All by itself, yogurt is a healthy green-light grow food, but most kinds of yogurt actually fall into the yellow-light category. A few even deserve to be downgraded to the red-light column. Here's a good label-reading lesson to share with your child. Look at the "yummy yogurt" label — the plain, unsweetened, unflavored yogurt. It lists two ingredients: milk and acidophilus, the "bugs," or bacteria, that turn the milk into yogurt and that also feed the growth of beneficial intestinal bacteria. Then check out some "yucky yogurts." Say, "Let's play I Spy! Do you detect any 'bad words' on the label?" When you check the ingredients list, you will see that many yogurts contain sweeteners, such as high-fructose corn syrup, and artificial colorings, such as red #40. Some have chemical sweeteners, such as sucralose and aspartame. These varieties have less protein and less calcium than plain yogurt. When they put the junky ingredients in, there is less room for the good stuff. Best nutritional solution? Buy the plain yogurt and add your own fruit at home. Thawed blueberries with their natural juices make a tasty flavoring for plain yogurt. Bananas and granola are good, too. If your child is accustomed to sweet yogurt, add a bit of honey (after one year of age) or pure maple syrup to make the plain yogurt more palatable at first.

Muscle foods. Jonathan was still itching to get back to the *Star Wars* aisle, so we headed there next because I needed some pictures of the enemy — the junk food. But on the way, we passed the meat section, so we stopped to talk about muscle foods. I explained to the kids that the slices of meat we were looking at were actually muscles of animals. We first looked at a big steak that was nicely marbled with fat. Cooked on the barbecue this would look pretty good, but in its raw state it was less appealing. I said, "See the muscle? The white stuff in it is fat. There's a lot of it in there. I wonder why." We talked about how this meat came from a steer and what this steer did all day. "This steer just stood around all day, didn't get to run, didn't get much exercise, and ate fattening food." We talked about how this is what our muscles would look like if we just sat around and watched TV or played video games all day, and how we wouldn't be very strong.

What seven-year-old boy wants to have weak muscles? Jonathan is always showing us how strong he is and how fast he can run. I suggested he look around for some better muscle foods. He found a piece of "meat" that had hardly any fat on it at all and wanted to know what kind of animal it came from. I saw that it was a big piece of salmon. I said, "Jonathan, this muscle came from something that got a lot of exercise. This came from a big fish that swam around all day. And this must be what your muscles look like, too, since you get lots of exercise. Right?" "Right!"

Then we talked about what this fish ate. "Jonathan, do you think this fish ate lots of ice cream and candy?" He knew the answer: "Of course not. Fish don't eat those things, Dad!" "Of course they don't, and look how healthy they are because of it!"

Wonderful waffles, awful waffles. We walked through the frozen foods section, looking for waffles. This supermarket stocks an increasing variety of healthy foods, as a way of competing with the specialty stores frequented by shoppers looking for alternatives to the standard American diet. There were several varieties that looked like healthy alternatives to the white-flour popular brands. These included whole-grain, flaxseed, and buckwheat waffles. I thought all of these waffles sounded pretty healthy, but I decided to check a few labels anyway. I was surprised to find big differences in the amounts of fat, sugar, protein, and fiber in the various brands. One brand had about twice as much sugar as another brand and not as much fiber, and this was the one with the more aggressive "healthy food" messages on the packaging. The words "flax" and "whole grain" were in large print on the front of the box, but the fine print in the Nutrition Facts box and the ingredients list told a different story. We left these waffles in the frozen food case and put the less flashy but nutritionally better brand in our cart.

My kids really like toaster waffles for breakfast, but we skip the usual pancake syrup, which is made from high-fructose corn syrup and contains an alarming amount of junk carbs. Instead, we encourage the kids to top their waffles with fruit and maybe

---

SHOPPING RULES FOR KIDS

Let your kids know the rules before you venture into the supermarket:

- We mainly shop the perimeter of the store.
- We buy whole grains.
- We buy mostly grow foods.
- We read labels carefully.
- We don't buy foods or beverages with "bad words" on the label.

just a touch of pure maple syrup. I have been surprised to discover that a large number of kids eat their waffles and pancakes without syrup. Kids seem to recognize that it's just too sweet and that syrupy waffles can leave them feeling icky.

Not-so-good grains. Well, we finally made it to the cereal aisle. I had no intention of buying cereal. I just wanted to look at it and take some pictures for my lecture. Of course, the kids really liked this aisle because it was filled with packages featuring *Star Wars* characters, Bugs Bunny, and Shrek, all concentrated at kids' eye level. So I told my kids that they could pick out any cereal they wanted, as long as the "sugar number" was 5 (about 1 teaspoon) or lower. A bit of "sugar" added is okay, as long as it is partnered with lots of protein and fiber. I showed them the line in the Nutrition Facts box for number of grams of sugar per serving. My son soon discovered that the Darth Vader cereal had 13 grams of sugar per serving! The box with the big white happy bunny on the front that promised a neat prize inside didn't fare any better. The sugar number was 13, with fiber and protein numbers of only 1 gram each! A child who eats this for breakfast and then goes off to school won't function well in a classroom for very long.

The kids soon found that there were only a few cereals on the shelf with an acceptable number, until we found something called Mighty Bites by Kashi. This cereal had a sugar number of 5 (which is good), a fiber number of 3 (pretty good for a kid cereal), and, to my delight, 5 grams of protein. In addition, I saw it was a whole-grain cereal. This was a perfect cereal for my kids. And it actually appealed to the kids. The package showed real kids playing and looking like they were growing and having fun. Ah! A grow food message instead of a movie character on the box. It passed the final test at home — it tasted really good.

Jonathan then eyed some smaller boxes across the aisle that

GREEN-LIGHT CEREALS

As you cautiously venture into the cereal section, where there are many label lessons, play I Spy again. Lead your child to the "green-light cereals." Have them look for these ingredients:

- whole grains, not just wheat; preferably "100% whole grain"
- at least 5 grams of protein per serving
- at least 3 grams of fiber per serving
- less than 6 grams of added sugar per serving
- no added artificial sweeteners (e.g., high-fructose corn syrup)
- no "bad words" (e.g., red #40, hydrogenated oils)
- bonus: added iron, calcium, zinc, vitamins, folate, DHA, probiotics

---

also had Darth Vader on them. I said, "Okay, let's look at the back, Jonathan, and see if this would be a good breakfast. What's the sugar number?" It was 18, three times Dad's limit. And that was just for a small serving. Many people eat much more. Definitely not the way to start the day. (For why not, see page 190.) Darth Vader was definitely a bad influence.

Bread basics. The bread aisle was next. My kids usually take sandwich lunches to school, so they eat bread every day. They resist the thick, whole-grain-sprouted breads that are so good for them, and, like most kids, prefer lighter, whiter, fluffier bread. I am determined to change their tastes. We first grabbed a familiar brand, which I will not name (however, I do "wonder" why so many parents buy it), and then selected another loaf made from whole and even sprouted grains. I asked Lea to hold one in each hand and to compare them. She quickly noticed that one was much heavier than the other. I said, "I wonder why. What do you think?" She looked at the breads and said, "Well, this heavier bread feels a lot thicker. There probably aren't as many bubbles in the bread." I asked her, "What's inside a bubble?" She said, "Air. This light bread must be full of air." I asked her, "Do you think eating a lot of air gives you much energy for school?" and she giggled and said, "Of course not, Daddy. That's silly."

I asked Lea to look at the heavy bread and to tell me what she saw. "Well, Daddy, I see some seeds. This bread looks a lot darker than the other bread, and it's not at all squishy." Seizing the moment, I asked Jonathan, "Do you want your muscles to feel squishy like the air bread or strong like the grow bread?"

We talked about why the "seeds" are so good for you. "These seeds are the grains that flour is made from. With lighter breads, the grains are all crushed, and the good brown outside part is taken out, leaving just a white powder, which is called flour. This flour is used to make a fluffy white bread that's full of bubbles. But if you crush up the grains and put ALL of it — the powder and the good brown part — into the flour you use to make the bread, it's much better for you and gives you lots of energy." Lea thought she might like to try some healthy bread, so we found one that looked pretty good to both of us and brought it home for sandwiches. I asked her the next day if she had liked her turkey sandwich with the healthy bread. She said, "I didn't think I would like it, but it was good." Once again I saw the importance of having kids help pick out the good foods.

Junky juice. My kids don't get much juice, so they were hoping for a special treat when we got to the juice aisle. It had almost as many cartoon characters as the cereal aisle, all calling out, "Hey, kids! Pick me! Pick me!"

Parents often ask me how much juice their children should

have. My answer is usually "The less they drink, the healthier they will be." Most "juice drinks" are mainly sugar water, with flavorings and colorings and perhaps a small amount of real fruit juice. Most kids get too much sugar as it is. They would be better off drinking water or milk, which offers protein and healthier sugars.

IS IT REAL JUICE?

Juice makers are very sneaky when it comes to labeling. A label may say "Made with All-Natural Fruit" or "Contains Pure Fruit Juices," and it wouldn't be lying. There is fruit or fruit juice in the product. But in fact, it contains mostly sugar, water, and artificial colors. Just because a juice is *made with* something natural doesn't mean there aren't other ingredients added. A juice whose label says "100% Pure, All-Natural Juice" contains just that. Confused? You're not alone. I usually don't trust the label on the front when it comes to juice. I read the actual ingredients on the back before I buy it.

Even juice that is "100 percent juice" doesn't offer a whole lot of nutrition. Juice is not crushed-up fruit. It's fruit with all the fiber removed. All that's left is the water, the fruit sugar, and the vitamins (some of which are destroyed in the processing). Eating an apple or a pear has tremendous nutritional value. You get fiber, vitamins, and carbs for energy; but if you drink the apple juice or pear juice without the fiber, you're getting a lot of sugar, with nothing to slow the absorption of these sugar carbs. It may be a "natural" sugar rush, but it's still a sugar rush. That's why juice is considered a treat in our house. As treats go, it's a healthy one, but it's not an everyday food. Jonathan, Lea, and I found some small bottles of 100 percent juice in the refrigerated section and decided this would be one of the special treats we bought on this shopping trip.

GO FOR GOOD BARS

Children enjoy snack bars for good grazing, and they can be a healthy alternative to candy bars. Instead of succumbing to the temptation of the junk bars at the checkout counter, take your child for a treat at the energy bar section. Green-light bars enjoy a similar nutrient composition to green-light cereals. Besides having a healthy protein and fiber composition (try for 5 grams of protein, 3 grams of fiber) and no "bad words" on the label, the best bars are sweetened with fruits, such as figs and dates. Beware of bars sweetened with corn syrup.

Getting out of the store. On the way to the checkout lanes, Jonathan spotted more boxes with Darth Vader on them and immediately said, "Daddy, I want that." "Well, what is it?" I asked. He said, "I don't know." We looked more closely at the box. It was snack crackers, and the Nutrition Facts box told us that they were full of hydrogenated fats and sodium. Jonathan knew not to pursue it. Whew! It's really nice to let the label itself say no; now I don't have to be the bad guy all the time.

We purchased some healthy food on this shopping trip, including bread, fruits and vegetables, and a good cereal. But it was very frustrating for me to listen to my kids clamor for foods that were not good for them. They were bombarded with messages encouraging them to make bad food choices, and I had to keep saying, "no, no, NO!"

LESSONS IN LABEL READING

If you want to know exactly what is in a particular package of food on the supermarket shelf, skip the hype on the front and look at the Nutrition Facts box on the back or side. This box is prepared by the food company, but its contents and how they are presented must meet requirements set by the U.S. Department of Agriculture. The Nutrition Facts box presents nutritional information in a standard format that makes it easier for consumers to compare products and to find out more about what they are buying.

Nutrition Facts

Serving Size	1 cup (33g/1.2 oz.)
Children Under 4	½ cup (17g/0.6 oz.)
Servings Per Container	About 9
Children Under 4	About 17

Amount Per Serving	Cereal	Cereal for Children Under 4
Calories	120	60
Calories from Fat	15	5
	% Daily Value	
Total Fat 1.5g	2%	0.5g
Saturated Fat 0g		0g
Trans Fat 0g		0g
Cholesterol 0mg		0mg
Sodium 160mg	7%	85mg
Potassium 110mg	3%	55mg
Total Carbohydrate 23g	8%	12g
Dietary Fiber 3g	12%	1g
Sugars 5g		3g
Other Carbohydrate 15g		8g
Protein 5g		3g

Serving Size. The box lists a standard serving size, and the information that follows is based on that size serving. Your idea of a serving may not be the same as the size listed on the box. For example, what you think of as "bowlful" of cereal may be more than the ¾ cup standard serving.

Calories. The box tells you how many calories are in a serving and how many of these calories come from fat. Depending on the type of fat, a high proportion of calories from fat may be a bad sign. Remember to adjust the number of calories (and other nutrient amounts, too) in a serving if your idea of a serving size is different from the one stated on the box.

% Daily Value. The next part of the box lists the amounts of fat, carbs, protein, and other nutrients in the food. It also tells what percentage of your daily need for a given nutrient is supplied by the food. Since there is no established daily value for protein, you won't find a percentage for protein on this line. The percentage of daily values are based on the 2,000-calorie diet of the average adult, so amounts for younger kids will differ, based on their calorie intake.

Total Fats. The box gives you a figure for total fat in a serving. It also tells you how much of that fat is saturated fat and, thanks to new labeling laws, how much is trans fats. (Funny, now that manufacturers must tell consumers about the amount of trans fats in their products, trans fats seem to be disappearing from many snack foods.) The box also gives you the amount of cholesterol present in one serving.

Total Carbohydrate. This line tells you the total number of grams of carbs from all sources, including the carbs naturally occurring in the food, plus the carbs (usually sugar or other sweeteners) added by the manufacturer.

Sugars. Here's where carb labeling gets confusing. "Sugars," under carbohydrates, include the naturally present sugars, including the fructose in fruit and the lactose in dairy foods, plus the sugars added to the food, such as corn syrup and table sugar. It would be more informative to label readers to have the term "added sugars," which would represent only those sugars added by the manufacturer.

For cereals, the Sugars line does refer to the number of grams of added sweetener. Here's a cereal label-reading tip for doing the math: the greater the discrepancy between Total Carbohydrates and Sugars, the more nutritious the cereal is likely to be. As you can see from the examples below, the Healthy Puffs has 23 grams of total carbohydrates and 5 grams of sugars. The Junky Puffs contains 28 grams of total carbs and 15 grams of sugars.

HEALTHY PUFFS			JUNKY PUFFS		
Nutrition Facts			**Nutrition Facts**		
Calories		120	**Calories**		120
Total Fat		1.5g	**Total Fat**		1.5g
Saturated Fat		0g	Saturated Fat		0g
Trans Fat		0g	*Trans* Fat		0g
Total Carbohydrate		23g	**Total Carbohydrate**		28g
Dietary Fiber		3g	Dietary Fiber		0.6g
Sugars		5g	Sugars		15g
Protein		5g	Protein		1g
Whole grains, vitamins, and minerals. No artificial colorings, hydrogenated oils, or high-fructose corn syrup.			Corn, wheat, vitamins, minerals, high-fructose corn syrup, artificial colorings, hydrogenated oils.		

Other Carbohydrate. This line tells you the number of grams of carbs in the grains themselves, not including the fiber but including nondigestible stabilizers.

Ingredients. At the bottom of the Nutrition Facts box, you'll find the ingredients in the food, listed from greatest amount by weight to the smallest. Here's where to look for those twin evils, hydrogenated fats and high-fructose corn syrup. This is an important list for parents of allergic kids, since eggs, cow's milk, wheat, corn, nuts, soy, and other allergenic substances can appear in all kinds of unexpected places.

SHOPPING FOR WHOLE FOODS

A few days later we made a trip to our local Whole Foods Market. What a difference! The first thing we saw when we entered the store was the produce section, full of beautifully displayed fruits and vegetables in a whole rainbow of colors. Darth Vader was nowhere to be found. To my surprise, the kids were wide-eyed, looking at all these colorful, healthy foods. They quickly found their favorite fruits, apples, bananas, and cantaloupe. I was delighted to see my kids being bombarded with good food messages.

Hooray for hummus! We spent some time looking through the items in the deli case. There were many different kinds of hummus. Hummus is made from chickpeas crushed into a paste and flavored with garlic, sweet peppers, and olive oil. It's a healthy dip for sliced vegetables or a spread for crackers. Hummus is part of one of our favorite lunches, which we call turkey rollups. We take a whole-grain tortilla, spread some hummus on it, maybe some guacamole, layer a few slices of turkey and some cheese, and then roll it up tightly. This is a fun food that the kids like to eat for lunch, and they can make it themselves.

Healthy hot dogs. We also saw some hot dogs in this section. Now, everyone knows hot dogs are not a healthy food. For one thing, they have a very high animal fat content. They also contain nitrates, which have been linked to an increased risk of pancreatic cancer and leukemia. Leukemia is my biggest fear when it comes to my own children (or anyone's children), so it is very easy for me to say NO to hot dogs. (Nitrates give hot dogs and other deli meats their pink color. The USDA actually tried to get these substances banned from our food supply in the 1970s, but the effort was blocked by the meat industry.) But surprise! The hot dogs we found in this deli case were nitrate free veggie dogs, so we bought these ones as a special treat.

Better breads. We soon made our way to the bread aisle. Most of the choices here were good. Using the "feel method," the kids picked up the different loaves and noticed that most of them were heavy. They chose some that tasted pretty good when we got them home. We even found a wheat-free bread for Lea to try, since we suspect that she may be experiencing a mild sensitivity to wheat. We also grabbed whole wheat hot dog buns to go with those healthy hot dogs.

Extra nutritious eggs. Next we looked at eggs. I showed the kids how to choose eggs that are enriched with DHA. DHA is an important omega-3 fat that is vital to a healthy immune system and a healthy brain. When you feed hens a diet enriched with DHA, you get eggs that have higher levels of DHA in them. If you compare a DHA egg with a regular egg, you will see that the DHA egg yolk is a darker yellow. To our minds, these eggs are worth the extra money. Usually, DHA-fed chickens are fed healthier diets in general, without antibiotics or growth hormones. Check the carton for more information about that.

Doubtful dairy. Milk is good for kids. It offers protein as well as milk sugar for energy, and it's a fill-up food. However, many cows are routinely fed antibiotics to keep them from getting sick, and hormones to increase their milk production. How this affects the humans who drink the milk is not known, so we choose to avoid this potential problem by buying organic cow's milk.

Many people don't tolerate milk very well — and they may not even know it. Kids with frequent tummyaches, headaches, chronic sniffles, or sore throats might feel much better after avoiding cow's milk for a while or trying goat's milk, which some persons digest easier. This is something I have noticed with many of my patients.

Safer seafood. Soon we came to the fish and meat section. We got to once again look at the difference between a fatty steak, of which there weren't a whole lot of examples in this store, and the salmon. We then noticed another big difference — there was an additional type of salmon that was even healthier-looking than the first one we had seen. What we were seeing was the difference between wild Pacific salmon and farmed Atlantic salmon. The wild salmon was a deeper, darker red than the farmed salmon. You can play Go Fish with your child. Show your child a piece of wild salmon (firm, dark pink, and with few fatty streaks). Compare it with a piece of farmed salmon (soft, pale, and with fatty streaks). Then say, "The strong fish ate grow food and swam hard upstream. The weak fish paddled in a pool all day and ate junk food. Which one do you think is which? Which fish would you like your muscles to be like?"

It's important to know where a fish comes from. Studies show that farmed salmon may contain unhealthy levels of mercury,

SHOPPING TIPS FROM DR. BILL

Maybe you like to shop with your kids. Maybe you don't. Either way, there will be days when you and your children go grocery shopping together. Here are some ways to get the job done.

- *Make a list.* A shopping list gives you a sense of purpose. It ensures that you will remember to buy the foods you need, and it keeps you from buying foods you don't need or want in your home. Enlist your children's help when you make your list. Tape a list of grow foods to your refrigerator and ask your children to check them off when they are used up so that you can add them to your shopping list. Ask your kids which grow foods they'd especially like, including, of course, a few acceptable treats. You might compare your shopping list with the traffic-light list on page 120. (Maybe you even have it posted on your refrigerator.) Be sure your shopping list contains mostly green-light grow foods, and perhaps a few yellow-light foods. Ignore the red-light foods.

- *Go directly to the grow foods.* As you enter the supermarket, say to your child, "We'll skip the junk-food aisles and go to the grow foods. Let's find the fruits and vegetables." Avoid dragging your kids past displays of stuff you're not going to buy.

- *Ask kids to help.* Kids love to bag apples, pick out lettuce, find foods on the shelves, and put things in the grocery cart. You could include pictures on your list of what to buy, or have your first-grader practice reading the words on your list.

- *Shop the perimeter.* Many stores are arranged with the produce, meat, and dairy foods around the perimeter of the store, and the more processed foods in the aisles in the middle. Stick to the outside for fresh foods and skip the junk-food and pop aisles.

- *Get away from "red-light" foods.* Besides saying, "We only shop the perimeter," tell your inquisitive child, "There is an aisle in the supermarket that we just don't go down." "Why?" she's likely to ask. "Because that aisle contains red-light foods, those with the three 'bad words' on the label: high-fructose corn syrup, hydrogenated oil, and a color with a number, like red #40."

- *Practice numbers and colors.* Kids can practice math and language skills at the supermarket. Count "one, two, three, four apples." Talk about what costs more and what costs less. Calculate prices per serving or per pound.

- *Just say no!* You can't get out of the store without going through the checkout lane, with all of its last-minute temptations. So prepare for last-minute appeals for candy by picking out healthier treats elsewhere in the store and handing them out while you wait in line. Remind your child, "We just don't eat that stuff in our family. Remember, we got you that special juice [or whatever] for a treat. For now, here's a handful of Mighty Bites [or whatever]."

PCB's, and other environmental pollutants. Wild Pacific salmon, on the other hand, is known to have much lower levels of pollutants, and therefore it is much healthier to eat, especially if you're going to eat it several times a week, like my dad does. He stays away from any farmed fish. My wife and I have decided that the wild salmon is the one to buy, even though it is a bit more expensive. It's well worth it for the food that's feeding our children's brains. Canned salmon is nearly always wild.

Taking it all home. Where and how you shop for food really does matter. I have discovered that the key to my family's eating healthy is to KEEP JUNK FOOD OUT OF THE HOUSE. Fill the pantry and refrigerator with only healthy choices, and then, when it comes time to make dinner or grab a snack, you have to make a healthy choice. If a hungry child (or adult) goes to the pantry looking for a snack, and both cookies and fruit are available, the cookies will win every time — guaranteed. Wise food choices need to be made while you're shopping, when you're not hungry. A pantry stocked with healthy snacks will ensure that your child is eating healthy most of the time. This actually makes it easier to say yes to the occasional junk treat, because you know your kids haven't already had two sodas, three juice boxes, and a bunch of cookies that day. Let home be a healthy eating zone. It may take a while for your family to get used to this, but they eventually will — mine did.

11

Common Nutrition Questions

GO ORGANIC

Are organic foods worth the extra money?

Yes! Your kids are worth it. I (Bill) was recently talking to a friend — and "pure parent" — about how good food leads to good growth and good performance. He replied, "I own a million-dollar racehorse and feed him the best food I can get. Certainly my children are more valuable than my horse." Pollutants in the air, in water, and in food all have the potential to harm your child's health. In addition to limiting your child's exposure to environmental toxins, give your child food that you know is free of pesticides and chemical fertilizers. Buying organic will help your kids be healthier.

Organic farming produces foods that you know are safe to feed your family. It also protects the air, soil, and water supply from potentially toxic pollutants. Organic produce is grown without pesticides, weed killers, and synthetic fertilizers. It is never genetically engineered or modified and is never irradiated.

When the label says "certified organic," it means that the food has been grown according to strict standards, and farm fields and processing facilities have been inspected to ensure that growers and packagers are meeting the regulatory standards for organic foods. Adults already have a significant body burden of environmental chemicals, which are almost impossible to get rid of. Your children have the chance to lead a "purer" life than you, at least when it comes to pesticides in foods. Organic foods are better for everyone, but they are probably more important to children's health than to adults'. Here are the reasons:

Growing bodies are more vulnerable. Rapidly growing and dividing cells, like those in growing children and pregnant women, are more susceptible to the carcinogenic risks of pesticides. Of course, the chemicals in food don't give you cancer all of a sudden. It's the repeated exposure and the buildup of these substances in the body that can lead to cancer and other illnesses.

Young bodies store more toxins. Pesticides are stored in fat, and young children, especially infants and toddlers, have proportionately more body fat than do adults — and thus more potential for storing toxins.

Adult "food safety limits" may not be safe for children. For government regulatory agencies to approve a pesticide for use on food crops, it must be designated "generally regarded as safe" (GRAS). The fact that a substance carries the GRAS label does not mean that the substance is definitely safe. Do you want to feed your family foods that are "generally" regarded as safe? There may be problems with the substance that haven't yet turned up in studies, often because the research has not looked at long-term exposure. You really don't know if a lifetime of exposure to a given pesticide will be okay for your children. Also, the maximum acceptable limits for how much of a substance is allowed in a food are based upon what is estimated to be safe for adults. But children do not eat or metabolize pesticides like little adults, and the amount of a food they eat is greater in proportion to their body weight than the same food eaten by an adult. A 25-pound child who eats a pesticide-laden peach is exposed to a relatively higher dose of the chemical than a 150-pound adult.

Safer foods are healthier foods. Organic food growers do not usually claim that organic foods are more nutritious than conventionally farmed foods, but studies are beginning to show that some organic foods contain higher levels of certain vitamins, minerals, and other nutrients. Some researchers believe that pesticides interfere with the plant's own immune system. It seems that plants grown without pesticides have a higher level of phytos (the germ fighters you learned about in chapter 8). This makes sense, since organic foods have to make more phytos to fight pests because they don't rely on pesticides to do it for them. So, they have a better opportunity to become the most nutritious tomato, carrot, or cabbage they can be.

We believe that families should choose organic food whenever possible, but limited food budgets and the availability of organic food may mean that it's not always possible to "go organic." Here are our suggestions for setting priorities and lessening your family's exposure to agricultural chemicals:

- *Buy the "dirty dozen" as organic.* Obviously, the fruits that are hard to clean or ones whose peels you eat are the most risky. Look for organic versions of the following:

apples	cantaloupe
apricots	cherries
blackberries	grapes

nectarines	raspberries
peaches	spinach
pears	strawberries

- *Buy organic dairy.* We believe strongly that children should not drink dairy products from cows that routinely receive growth hormones, antibiotics, and other less-than-natural substances.

- *Buy free-range, organic meat and poultry.* Some people feel that meat and poultry raised under more natural conditions, without antibiotics and hormones in their feed, are not only healthier but also taste better.

- *Buy organic dried fruit.* Dried fruits, such as raisins, prunes, and apricots, concentrate a large number of nutrients — and pollutants — in a small volume of food. You can find organic dried fruit in many nutrition-conscious markets.

- *Buy lean.* Choose lean meats and skim or low-fat milk, since pesticides tend to concentrate in fat.

VITAMIN AND MINERAL SUPPLEMENTS

How do I know if my child needs a multivitamin/multimineral supplement?

Growing children need more vitamins, minerals, and other nutrients per pound of body weight than do fully grown adults, but kids sometimes have erratic eating patterns and don't always eat the foods they should. Therefore, children are more likely than adults to have nutrient deficiencies. For this reason, many parents and pediatricians feel a daily vitamin and mineral supplement is like a nutritional insurance policy for children. Still, not every child needs vitamin supplements. Here are some things to consider:

- It's best to get nutrients from foods rather than from pills because, in a good example of *synergy,* many nutrients are absorbed better and work better in the body when they are consumed with other nutrient "friends." For example, iron is better absorbed if eaten with vitamin C–containing foods. Think iron-rich meatballs with the vitamin C in tomato sauce.

- There are hundreds of substances (and probably more to be discovered) in fruits and vegetables that boost health. You can't get all of them in vitamin supplements. Foods offer a wider, more healthful variety of nutrients than do pills.

- Vitamin and mineral supplements should not be used as an excuse to be less concerned about making healthy food habits a priority.

Kids with poor diets are the ones who need supplements most, yet they are the least likely to get them. Generally speaking, if you are interested enough in nutrition to want to read this book and if you follow the suggestions in it, your children probably don't need a multivitamin supplement.

The six most common nutrient deficiencies in children are omega-3 fats, iron, calcium, zinc, vitamin C, and vitamin E. You will see from the boxes below that it is not very difficult to get most of these nutrients from food sources.

Omega-3 fats. In our opinion, this is the number-one nutritional deficiency in children, since the standard American diet tends to be low in seafood and omega-3 rich fats. (See pages 98 and 171 for why children need omega 3's.) Unless your family eats a lot of cold-water fish, we suggest you give every family member a daily omega-3 supplement.

Iron. Kids need iron to make hemoglobin, the red component in the blood that carries oxygen to all the cells of the body. Iron is

HOW MUCH OMEGA-3 FAT DO YOU NEED EVERY DAY?

While there are no official government RDAs on the amount of daily omega-3 fats for children or adults, our recommendations are based on current research.

- children: ½ gram (500 mg) per day
- adults: 1 gram (1000 mg) per day

One gram means the total amount of omega-3 fatty acids. The most important two are DHA and EPA. The amount of these two omega 3's varies according to the brand, so you have to read the label carefully. Adults and pregnant and lactating women should aim for 400 milligrams of DHA and 600 milligrams of EPA daily. Infants and children should have around one-half this amount (200 mg. of DHA and 300 mg. of EPA). Children and adults who have neurological problems or mood disorders are often "treated" with four to six times these amounts.

BEST SOURCES OF OMEGA 3

Food	Omega-3 Fats (in grams)
Salmon (6 ounces)	2 to 3
Sardines (3 ounces)	2 to 3
Trout, rainbow (6 ounces)	2
Herring (3 ounces)	1.5
Tuna (6 ounces)	1 to 1.5
Halibut (6 ounces)	.8

As you can see, if you eat salmon two to three times a week, you will meet your average of *1 gram a day* requirement.

HOW MUCH IRON DO YOU NEED EVERY DAY?*

Children, 1 to 10 years	10 mg.
Adult males	10 mg.
Teen males	12 mg.
Teen and adult females	18 mg.
Pregnant women	30 mg.

* Average RDA (or DV, for daily values) for iron in milligrams

---

also a building block for neurotransmitters. A child with an iron deficiency has both a tired body and a tired brain. Preschool children are especially prone to iron-deficiency anemia, which is why your child's health-care provider may obtain a blood sample to measure hemoglobin levels during yearly checkups.

Calcium. Kids need calcium to build strong bones. Getting enough calcium in the early years lowers the risk of osteoporosis later in life. It's like putting nutritional money in the bank. Your investment goal is strong bones. Taking calcium supplements to build bone strength after bones are fully grown is not as effective as eating a calcium-rich diet during childhood when bones are growing. Calcium is also necessary for strong brains. It contributes to efficient neurotransmitter function.

It's not how much calcium is in the food that matters. The amount of that calcium that gets into your child's body is important. To boost calcium absorption:

- *Eat calcium-rich foods more frequently.* Calcium is best absorbed when taken in smaller amounts more frequently. (Another reason why grazing is good for you.)

BEST SOURCES OF IRON

Food	Iron (in milligrams)
Meat and Poultry	
Beef (4 ounces)	3.5
Ground beef (4 ounces)	2.5
Lamb (4 ounces)	2.5
Turkey (dark meat, 4 ounces)	2.5
Chicken (dark meat, 4 ounces)	1.6
Turkey (light meat, 4 ounces)	1.6
Veal (4 ounces)	1.5
Chicken (light meat, 4 ounces)	1.0
Pork (4 ounces)	1.0
Seafood	
Oysters (½ cup)	8.0
Clams (4 ounces)	3.0
Shrimp (4 ounces)	2.0
Tuna (3 ounces)	1.0
Vegetables	
Spirulina (1 tsp.)	5.0
Tomato paste (4 ounces)	3.9
Lentils (4 ounces)	3.0
Beet greens (1 cup)	2.7
Jerusalem artichokes (4 ounces)	2.5
Potato (with skin, 1)	2.5
Barley (4 ounces)	2.0
Beans (½ cup)	2.0
Chickpeas (½ cup)	2.0
Artichokes, raw (½ cup)	2.0
Pumpkin (4 ounces)	1.7

Food	Iron (in milligrams)
Sauerkraut (4 ounces)	1.7
Sweet potatoes (4 ounces)	1.7
Tomato purée (4 ounces)	1.1
Peas (4 ounces)	1.0
Tomato sauce (4 ounces)	0.8
Potato (without skin, 1)	0.6

Grains and Cereals

Grains for baking (amaranth and quinoa)	8.0 to 9.0
Cream of Wheat (4 ounces)	5.0
Breakfast cereals (iron-fortified, 1 ounce)	4.0 to 8.0
Bagel (1 ounce)	1.8
Pasta (4 ounces)	1.0 to 2.0
Bread (whole wheat, 1 slice)	1.0

Fruits and Juices

Peaches, dried (6 halves)	3.1
Prune juice (8 ounces)	3.0
Figs (5)	2.0
Apricots, dried (10 halves)	1.6
Raisins (4 ounces)	1.5

Others

Chili con carne with beans (1 cup)	4.0
Pumpkin seeds (1 ounce)	4.0
Blackstrap molasses (1 tbsp.)	3.5
Infant formula (iron-fortified, 8 ounces)	3.0
Tofu, firm (3 ounces)	2.0 to 7.0
Sunflower seeds (1 ounce)	1.9
Brewer's yeast (1 tbsp.)	1.4
Nuts (almonds, peanuts, 1 ounce)	1.0

HOW MUCH CALCIUM DO YOU NEED EVERY DAY?

Infants (birth to 1 year)	400 to 600 mg.
Children (1 to 10 years)	800 mg.
Preteens and teens	1,200 to 1,500 mg.
Adults	1,200 mg.
Seniors	1,500 mg.
Pregnant or breastfeeding	1,500 to 2,000 mg.

BEST SOURCES OF CALCIUM

Best Dairy Sources	Calcium (in milligrams)
Yogurt, nonfat, plain (1 cup)	450
Yogurt, low-fat, plain (1 cup)	400
Parmesan cheese (1 ounce)	336
Romano cheese (1 ounce)	302
Milk, low-fat (1 cup), organic	300
Cheddar cheese (1 ounce)	200
Cottage cheese (1 cup)	155

Best Nondairy Sources	Calcium (in milligrams)
Sardines (3 ounces)	371
Orange juice, calcium-fortified (1 cup)	300
Sesame seeds (1 ounce)	280
Tofu (3 ounces)	190
Salmon (3 ounces, canned)	180
Collards (½ cup, chopped)	180
Rhubarb (½ cup)	174
Blackstrap molasses (1 tbsp.)	172

- *Eat calcium-rich foods with foods that contain vitamin C.* Citrus fruits and juices are good sources of calcium. Vitamin C improves calcium absorption, just as it does with the absorption of iron. Drink a glass of orange juice (or, better, eat an orange) with milk and cereal for breakfast or make a salad of fresh tomatoes and cottage cheese for lunch.

- *Avoid soft drinks.* Sodas contain citric or phosphoric acid (sodas used to be called "phosphates"), which can leach calcium from the bones and lessen the absorption. A 12-ounce can of the fizzy

Best Nondairy Sources	Calcium (in milligrams)
Amaranth flour (½ cup)	150
Spinach (½ cup, canned)	136
Figs (5)	135
Artichoke (1 medium)	135
Soybean nuts (¼ cup)	116
Cereal, calcium-fortified (½ cup)	100 to 200
Turnip greens (½ cup, chopped)	100
Kale (½ cup, chopped)	90
Almond butter (2 tbsp.)	86
Beet greens (½ cup, boiled)	82
Almonds (1 ounce)	80
Bok choy (Chinese cabbage) (½ cup)	79
Okra (½ cup)	77
Tempeh (½ cup)	77
Beans (½ cup, baked)	75
Papaya (1 medium)	73
Orange (1 medium)	50
Broccoli (½ cup, chopped)	47

stuff can rob the body of 100 milligrams of calcium. Drinking lots of soda is like robbing the child's calcium bank.

Zinc. Zinc is often overlooked as an important mineral, and many children don't get enough. Zinc strengthens the immune system and is used to make enzymes that are necessary for cell division and optimal growth. Like omega 3's, calcium, and iron, zinc also has a role in optimal brain function.

HOW MUCH ZINC DO YOU NEED EVERY DAY?

Children (1 to 10 years)	10 mg. per day
Adults	15 mg. per day

BEST SOURCES OF ZINC

Food	Zinc (in milligrams)
Crab (3 ounces)	7.0
Beef (lean, 3 ounces)	6.0
Turkey (dark meat, 3 ounces)	4.0
Wild rice (¼ cup, dry)	3.0
Wheat germ (¼ cup)	2.5
Tofu (½ cup, firm)	2.0
Yogurt (8 ounces, plain)	2.0
Artichoke (1 medium)	1.5
Nuts (1 ounce)	1.4
Oatmeal (¼ cup, dry)	1.3
Chickpeas (½ cup, canned)	1.3
Cereals, zinc fortified (1 ounce)	1.0 to 10.0
Beans: kidney, lima (½ cup)	0.75

Vitamin E. Vitamin E has gotten a lot of attention as a nutrient that protects the heart and brain from the effects of aging. Yet it is often overlooked as a vitamin needed by growing children. Vitamin E is an important antioxidant. It helps children develop a

---

HOW MUCH VITAMIN E DO YOU NEED EVERY DAY?

Children (1 to 10 years)	10 to 30 IU*
Adults	30 IU

* IU stands for "international units." It's difficult to determine the optimal dosage of these nutrients for every child, since the RDA's are based on an "average" need and are considered by many nutritionists to be like a minimum wage, the lowest level to prevent disease but perhaps not enough to promote optimal wellness.

BEST SOURCES OF VITAMIN E

Food	Vitamin E (in International Units, or IU)
Wheat germ oil (1 tbsp.)	26
Sunflower seeds (1 ounce)	21
Nuts (1 ounce)	10
Wheat germ, raw (2 tbsp.)	4
Vitamin E–enriched cereals	3 to 7
Nut oils (1 tbsp.)	3 to 6
Potato skins	3 to 5
Peanut butter (2 tbsp.)	3
Spinach (1 cup)	3
Tomato paste (¼ cup)	3
Seafood (6 ounces)	2 to 3
Avocado (1 medium)	3
Blueberries (1 cup)	2

strong immune system, protects cell membranes from damage, reduces inflammation in blood vessels, and plays an important role in cholesterol metabolism and the formation of healthy blood cells.

Antioxidants. Antioxidants (see page 184) are relative newcomers to the supplement field. There are no *research-based* recommended intakes for the different types of antioxidants for children or adults. Nevertheless, these are important nutrients. Fruits and vegetables are the richest sources of antioxidants. Vitamins E and C are potent antioxidants. New studies suggest the daily need for vitamin C to promote optimal wellness is far above the RDA of 60 milligrams per day. We believe the range to shoot for is 250 to 500 milligrams per day. Following the USDA's recommendation of nine servings of fruits and vegetables, children and adults would get this amount.

BEST SOURCES OF VITAMIN C

Food	Vitamin C (in milligrams)
Sweet pepper, yellow or green, 1 medium	240
Guava, 1 medium	165
Chili pepper, 1 large	109
Papaya, 1 cup, cubed	87
Strawberries, 1 cup	84
Orange, 1 medium	75
Kiwi, 1 medium	74
Cantaloupe, 1 cup	68
Broccoli, ½ cup, lightly steamed	41

SOURCES OF SUPPLEMENTS

As of this writing, the supplement industry is in a state of flux because of changes being made in research-based recommendations for appropriate doses of vitamins and minerals. Please consult our website, AskDrSears.com/supplements, for the latest information on vitamin and mineral supplements for children, especially dosages and our current recommendations.

VEGGIE TIPS

I know vegetables are good for my children, but they don't like them. Help!

Helping your children learn to like vegetables is one of the most valuable health gifts you can give them. It may take some time and effort to get your children to appreciate a wide variety of vegetables, but it's worth it.

Veggies are grow foods. Vegetables are nutrient dense. They pack a lot of nutrition into relatively few calories. Kids like variety in food, and veggies come in many varieties.

Veggies are health foods. Vegetables are Mother Nature's pharmacy. Their rich colors signal the presence of powerful phytonutrients, like the following:

- Red veggies (tomatoes, bell peppers) deliver the antioxidant lycopene.

- Orange and yellow veggies (sweet potatoes, pumpkin, carrots, squash) contain both beta carotene and vitamin C.

- Greens (spinach, broccoli, green peppers, romaine lettuce) have lots of beta carotene, folate, and vitamin C.

- Dark red kidney beans and black beans are rich in vitamins, minerals, and phytos.

Veggies are lean foods. Vegetables are a boon for overeaters. You can fill your stomach with high-fiber vegetables while taking in relatively few calories — and you burn many of those calories chewing and digesting what you've eaten. That's why we call veggies "free foods" and "green-light foods."

Veggies are feel-good foods. The balance of good carbs, fiber, and some protein in vegetables, especially legumes, leave you with a good gut feeling and steady blood sugar levels.

Tips to Grow a Veggie Lover

Some vegetables have strong flavors that children find it hard to appreciate. Some have textures that kids need to get used to. It takes patience and ingenuity to market vegetables to picky eaters. But if you keep trying and make vegetables fun, kids will come around.

Grow your own veggies. Plant a vegetable garden. Kids are more likely to eat foods they grow and care for. Personalize the plants. If Susan helps you sow the seeds, the plant and its products become "Susan's squash."

> *Henry enjoys planting his seeds in the garden and watching them grow and then eating his bounty. I'm not sure he would eat so much arugula if he hadn't planted it himself. This makes him an adventuresome eater.*

◆

When my son was younger, we planted pole beans which grew on a lattice that leaned against the house. The vines went everywhere, and you had to search out the beans. They were fun to watch, fun to pick, and even fun to eat. (Be sure to pick them when they're young and tender, not old and tough.)

Take a veggie trip. During the growing season, take your children vegetable picking at a nearby farm or veggie patch. If you live in an urban area, find a farmer's market, where farmers bring their produce to a street corner or parking lot to sell. Farmer's markets are fun, festive places to shop and have an astounding array of fresh fruits and vegetables. Call the veggie patch "Mother Nature's *Farm*acy."

We started giving veggies fun names, like "little trees" (broccoli), "scary Gus" (asparagus), "arty-chokes" (artichokes), and "rabbit food" for salads.

"In our family, we eat vegetables." Surround your children with veggies: bowls of tomatoes, peppers, and so forth. Serve them at every meal — cooked, raw, plain, fancy, with dips and sauces, as part of casseroles, and as main dishes. Letting your children know that you consider vegetables to be a tasty part of every meal will help them form the habit of eating vegetables.

A couple nights a week I put out my son's "special plate," his Elmo plate, filled with cut-up veggies.

Market veggies. Put the foods you most want your children to eat within arm's reach. Keep a tray of cut-up veggies handy in the re- frigerator. Set it out on the counter or table when children nose around the kitchen for a snack before dinner. Cut them into in- teresting shapes: radish roses, cucumber wheels (take off strips of peel so the cukes are green-and-white striped), and celery sticks with fringed ends. Kids are often so fascinated with the interesting shapes that they overlook the fact that what they are eating are vegetables. Kitchen stores and catalogs have lots of ideas for making vegetables look good, and kids appreciate the fuss.

I keep fruits and veggies in a low place in the fridge, where they are easily accessible. I prewash them and sometimes fill snack bags with a portion for each child. I let my children have fruits and veggies as often as they want, any time they want, throughout the day.

Make veggies fun and tasty. Steaming preserves the color and flavor of vegetables. Drizzle them with olive oil or cover them with your child's favorite melted cheese. Spice veggies up with lemon or lime juice, oregano, basil, or garlic. Sweeten the taste with cinnamon, raisins, or honey.

My daughter loves raw, sweet "onion rings" on her fingers.

Make veggies nonthreatening. Some children may be more willing to eat vegetables if you cook them more rather than less. Foods such as broccoli and cauliflower are easier to chew and have a more mellow flavor if they are boiled rather than steamed. Trim away any tough fibrous parts. Yes, this makes the veggie a little less nutritious, but if your child won't eat the lightly steamed, still-crunchy broccoli, he won't get any nutritional value from it at all. Consult a good cookbook for ideas. Children may be more accepting of vegetables if you concentrate less on the virtues of eating veggies and more on flavor.

I hold back some of the regular-portion size of what my child really likes, such as any form of chicken, and tell her that she can have more after she eats a certain number of bites of veggies.

Sweeten veggies with fruit. Add Craisins (dried cranberries) to a spinach salad. Mix cooked apples with a cooked hard-shell squash such as butternut. Make a salad of romaine and citrus slices, either grapefruit or oranges, and serve with a honey-sweetened dressing.

Hide veggies. For the hard-core reluctant veggie eater, you may have to resort to tricks. Camouflage veggies chopped fine in pasta dishes, vegetable soup, tomato sauce, and stir-fries. Or cover them with sauce. Puréed veggies (e.g., carrots) "disappear" in spaghetti sauce. Our children liked "cheese in trees" (broccoli florets covered with melted cheddar). For more hide-the-veggies tricks, see Sneaky Tips to Get Nutrients into Your Family's Food, page 130.

We make a fruit-and-veggie smoothie about four parts fruit to one part vegetable, so the kids taste less of the veggies.

◆

I use my food processor to finely chop broccoli and other veggies, then add them to spaghetti sauce and other saucy foods. When the veggies are added in small amounts (which can be increased over time), my kids don't even realize the veggies are in there.

Let your kids cook. Encourage your children to help you prepare the vegetables. Kids love to pour and stir. Show them how to skewer vegetable kabobs. Vegetable pizza is a proven winner.

Use peer pressure. Invite over some vegetable-loving kids for a veggie party and watch your child copy what they eat.

Make a veggie roll-up. Roll a tortilla around veggies (instead of meat) and cheese. Fill a whole-wheat pita pocket with diced, cooked vegetables and add some hummus or yogurt.

Make veggie dips. Kids like to dip. Hummus, guacamole, tomato sauce, refried beans, puréed pumpkin, and yogurt seasoned with curry powder are favorite dips for broccoli florets (steamed or raw), sliced bell peppers, cherry tomatoes, and carrots (cooked or raw).

Serve veggie snacks. One of our favorite "nutri-tricks" was to serve our children veggies when they were the most hungry. Try putting cut-up veggies in a plastic bag for traveling or sporting events.

> *I give my daughters a bowl of cooked green beans or edamame to nibble on about forty-five minutes before dinner when they are watching a video while I cook. When they are getting hungry, they are more willing to eat whatever is handed to them. I give them the same kind of things to eat in the car, another great captive-audience time.*

Make a veggie lunch. A meal that helps get plenty of raw veggies into your kids' diet is lunch. Children love to help cut veggies up, and when they've made and arranged lunch for everyone, veggies are even more appealing. Try carrots, celery, cucumber, broccoli, and apples chopped up, served with nut butter, hummus, or a healthy homemade bean dip. It's finger food and fun to eat! This kind of lunch is easy to prepare and a good source of energy and nutrients, without the heaviness of cooked food.

Make veggie art. Using a whole-wheat tortilla, a pancake, or a circle of pizza dough as a base, let children create colorful faces with vegetables. Our kids' favorite: zucchini pancakes with a guacamole beard, olive eyes, tomato ears, carrot nose, bell-pepper mustache, blueberry hair, and a green bean smile. (See also Pretty Pizza, page 307.)

Serve veggie burgers. Kids love a burger, but it doesn't have to always be made of meat. Try veggie burgers for variety. Serve them in hamburger buns (whole wheat, of course) with the usual trimmings. Tomato, onion, guacamole, and leaf lettuce on a soy burger is a lot of veggies in a bun. When camouflaged with the child's favorite toppings, veggie burgers can taste like a hamburger.

Play veggie games. Make up games to encourage young children to eat vegetables. Name your child's favorite character from a book or television show and claim that that character likes veggies ("Nemo likes carrots and broccoli"). Eating vegetables is more fun when an imaginary character is eating them, too. If your child is going through a "mine" phase, tease him a bit by grabbing a veggie off his plate. He's likely to protest and say "mine" and reflexively take a bite.

Trains, planes, and "Star Wars" bites. Even our own kids have gone through picky phases. Dr. Bob found one way he could always ensure his kids took a few bites of veggies at dinnertime:

> *All my kids are big* Star Wars *fans. (I wonder who they got that from?) When they were younger, if they were in a finicky mood, I would turn their veggies into* Star Wars *ships flying around on my fork. They would play the role of the "giant space worm that loves to gobble up ships." For those of you who don't let your kids watch violent space movies, old-fashioned airplanes or choo-choo trains work great, too.*

Here are some other tricks parents have shared with us:

> *For our three-year-old we would say, "Rabbit, stay out of Mr. McGregor's garden!" Every time she would laugh and reach for the veggies on her plate.*

◆

I use the counting game with my son, since he's into counting every-thing he stacks or sees or moves. When I give him beans or peas, I always make a big deal out of counting them as I put them on his tray. He becomes so fascinated with my counting that he begins to count them, too, and eventually he counts what he eats.

◆

Jake likes taking the stems off the organic strawberries, which we call "removing their hats." We call baby carrots "logs rolling across a plate" with broccoli florets and asparagus "trees." Jake eats the whole "treetop" all at once.

◆

We have a game we call the new-taste game. Our daughter is three years old, so we give her a choice: "You can choose the broccoli, the chicken, or the beets for your new taste."

◆

I give Stephen the number of veggies to fit his age, such as nine green beans.

◆

We get the food to talk to our child: "No, don't eat me! Ouch!" This coming from a carrot has persuaded my obstinate four-year-old to eat the poor thing.

◆

I serve veggies with toothpick "swords" that my son uses to stab them.

EATING HEALTHY WHEN EATING OUT

We like to go out to restaurants. How can I encourage my children to order the healthy stuff on the menu and stay away from the junk?

Going out to eat can be healthy and fun, if you know where to go and what to eat when you get there. Here are some tips on keep-ing your kids on track while eating out.

Select kid-friendly restaurants. Choose restaurants that fit your family's healthier style of eating. These are the ones that offer salad bars with green greens, whole-grain breads, and healthy choices on the menu. Look for restaurants that focus on quality rather than large portions of foods that feature junk carbs and unhealthy fats. If you have to argue with your children about what they may choose from the menu, scratch the place off your list. Eating out should be a special treat that's fun, not an occasion for fights about food.

Fast-food restaurants target kids with their advertising, but that doesn't mean these are the only restaurants children will like. If your children pester you about eating at junk-food joints, invoke the "we" principle: "We just don't go there. That's not grow food." Enough said!

If you have a bright, inquisitive child who pesters you for junk food, play show-and-tell: Buy a chicken nugget at a junk-food outlet. Take it home and compare it with a homemade one. Tell your child, "The junk-food nugget is made with mashed-up chicken with a lot of junk chemicals added that are not grow foods. The chicken nugget that Mommy makes has only grow foods in it." Let him feel and taste the difference between the chemical food and the real food. Press both the nuggets to watch the bad oil come out of the junk one. He still may prefer the junk taste, but you can tell him *why* they make them taste so irresistible.

Pre-feed. If your kids can't control their appetites at restaurants — especially buffets — feed them a nutritious snack just before you leave home.

> *We decided to be more creative in celebrating an evening out on the town. We call our new tradition "dining in — and out." We begin by dressing up our children and inviting them to meet at our family*

SALAD SUGGESTIONS

Salads are a smart way to get a variety of veggies into kids. Try these salad-savvy tips:

- Frequent family-friendly restaurants that feature a salad bar with green greens like spinach and arugula, not just iceberg lettuce. In kid-think, salads are much cooler when served at restaurants. Salad bars offer a rainbow of colorful foods in shapes that kids love. Children enjoy creating their own combinations and arranging the food on their plate. Salad bars appeal to finicky eaters and kids who like to control their own food choices.

  We have a salad-bar night at home with lots of fresh cut-up fruits and veggies. For protein we add some tuna, chicken breast chunks, or blocks of tofu.

- Encourage kids to create their own salads at home. They will have fun designing their own.

  I have my children make individual salads to serve at lunch or dinner. I handle the parts that require a sharp knife and they assemble the salads. I ask them to be creative and "make a face" in each person's salad.

---

dining table. Candlelight adds a nice touch. Here the first course of fresh-cut vegetables and sliced fruit is served. Our three sons pick up on the excitement of the evening and fill their tummies with wonderful nourishment. We then travel to the restaurant for the entrée, being selective about ordering the most healthy offerings on the menu. Because we do not arrive at the restaurant in a state of excessive hunger, the children do not get restless while waiting for their food. They also tend to be more prudent about ordering smaller portions. We order water as a beverage. After enjoying this

They place lettuce on the plate, add some cherry tomatoes for the eyes, cucumber wedges for eyebrows, a carrot nose, and a strip of jicama for the teeth.

- Occasionally include a nutritious but less favorite food (e.g., tofu cubes) in your children's salad. Encourage them to try "one new food" in their familiar salad mixture.

- Use greens that are deep green, such as spinach, arugula, or romaine, instead of iceberg lettuce. The deeper the color, the more nutritious the leaf. Sweeten the greens with diced fruits, such as raisins or blueberries.

- Serve a satisfying salad at the beginning of the meal to curb the appetite of the compulsive overeater.

- Play dress-up. After they arrange their veggies in cute designs on top of the salad greens, encourage your children to experiment with nutritious dressings, such as hummus, olive oil and balsamic vinegar, and homemade honey-mustard dressing.

(See Dr. Bill's Super Salad recipe, page 308.)

stage of the meal, we return home for the final course. Ready and waiting is a homemade, whole-food dessert, such as apple crisp baked with fresh honey from our family's own beehives.

Go ethnic. Try new cuisines when you dine out with your children. Make eating out an exciting and novel event, not just a convenient way to eat food they can get at home. This is a creative way to get your children to try new foods.

Our kids love Japanese restaurants. They love to watch their food being prepared, and they have fun using the chopsticks. They seem to enjoy the theatrics so much that they are willing to try new foods.

Order grow foods before fun foods. Make it a rule that children must eat grow foods before fun foods. Tell your children, "It's okay to have dessert, but let's be sure we have something nutritious first." Try these ordering tips:

- *Scratch the kids' menus.* Kids' menus are filled with some of the junkiest foods around — hot dogs, breaded and processed chicken, processed french fries. Restaurant owners assume that kids are happy to eat junk foods and parents are happy to let them. If the restaurant's regular menu fits your family's eating values, ask the hostess to skip the kids' menus. Or, with older kids, compare the kids' menu to the adult menu and guide them to the healthier choices. Show them how kids' menus have limited choices and junk foods. Tell them that just because they're kids doesn't mean they don't deserve better food.

- *Eat salad or soup first.* Choose a restaurant that has a salad bar. Soups and/or salads keep your child from wanting the white bread. Ask your waiter ahead of time not to bring it to your table.

- *Ask for smaller portions from the adult menu.* Either ask for a smaller portion for your child (for a smaller price) or let your children share an adult portion.

- *Offer choices.* As you look at the menu together, point out three or four healthy choices and let your child select what she will eat. For kids, part of the fun of going out is having more control over what they eat than they do at home. If your child wants to order something that you don't want her to have, offer an alternative: "Instead of french fries you can order fresh fruit or salad." "Instead of a soda, choose water with lemon or the all-juice drink listed here."

For special occasions, like an older child's birthday, a soft drink could be chosen and would really stand out when the usual fare is water.

Grill the waiter — about the quality of food. The waiter is there to answer questions about the food, so ask about how the meat or fish is prepared (e.g., what kind of oil the restaurant uses). Request whole-grain bread, broiled or grilled entrées, sauces and salad dressings on the side, and olive oil in place of butter. Most restaurants will be happy to accommodate you.

Try novel feeding tricks. Let your children do things that they don't routinely do at home, such as use the restaurant-supplied toothpicks as spears for their peas, beans, and other spearable foods.

PROBIOTICS

I've been hearing a lot about probiotics. What are they, and do my children need them?

Very popular in Europe, probiotics are gaining acceptance in America. Probiotics, or "bowel bugs," as they are sometimes called, are healthful bacteria that reside in the colon normally. In return for a warm place to live, they do good deeds in the gut. The best-known probiotic is lactobacillus acidophilus, the familiar bacteria in popular probiotic foods such as yogurt, miso (soybean paste), and kefir (liquid yogurt).

Probiotics keep harmful bacteria in check. The gut is home to billions of bacteria, good and bad. The good bacteria colonize the gut and keep the bad bacteria from multiplying (hence the name "probiotic" or "pro-life"). When the harmful bacteria overtake the healthy ones, they cause inflammation and damage to the intestinal lining, which results in an upset stomach and/or diarrhea. Probiotics are helpful in preventing and treating any upset in the balance of bugs in the bowels.

Probiotics also convert the fiber in food to healthful fatty acids that nourish the cells lining the intestine. These short-chain fatty acids are also absorbed from the intestines into the liver, where they decrease the liver's production of cholesterol.

Here are some examples of situations in which a probiotic supplement may prove useful:

- Probiotics can help restore balance to the bacteria in the gut when you or your child must take an antibiotic to battle an infection. The antibiotic prescribed for your child's ear infection may kill not only the bacteria in the ear but also the good bacteria in the gut. This is why diarrhea is a common side effect of antibiotics. You can replenish the good bacteria with probiotics.

- Probiotics are part of the treatment regimen for chronic inflammatory bowel disease, such as colitis.

- Probiotics are often used to treat or prevent oral or vaginal yeast infections or urinary tract infections.

Probiotics have a terrific track record of safety. You can find them in yogurt (look for the words "live and active cultures" on the label). Probiotics are also available without prescription in capsule and powder form. In our pediatric practice, we frequently prescribe probiotics as preventive medicine. Probiotics help to protect toddlers and preschoolers from outbreaks of infectious diarrhea at day care.

Because probiotics don't live in the gut for a long time, they need to be replaced frequently. This is one of the reasons yogurt is on our list of superfoods. A cup of yogurt a day could be just what the doctor ordered to help your children enjoy intestinal health.

DIET DRINKS

Everyone in our family drinks soda, and we all are carrying a bit too much weight. Would it be helpful to switch to diet drinks?

No! While you are wise to look for ways to cut empty calories from your family's diet, switching from drinks sweetened with sugar or corn syrup to diet drinks is just substituting one harmful junk food for another. Sweeteners are the source of calories in soda and similar beverages. Using artificial sweeteners removes the calories, but these factory-made chemical sweeteners can be just as bad for the body, and for growing children, even worse. We have read the research on the safety of artificial sweeteners, especially aspartame and sucralose (see page 85), and we certainly wouldn't feed them to our children. We strongly advise you to exercise the same caution in your family.

Teach your children to drink water when they are thirsty, and model this behavior yourself. Keep a pitcher of water in the refrigerator — this makes water more interesting to kids. Substitute bottles of water for cans of soda in your pantry. To make flavored water, add a small amount of fruit juice or a slice of lemon or orange. Or make iced herbal tea in various fruit flavors. Remind your kids to carry a water bottle with them when they leave the house so that when thirst strikes, they won't be tempted by soda and other sweetened drinks.

SCHOOL MEALS

We eat healthy foods at home, but our children are exposed to so much junk food at school. What can we do?

We often give nutrition talks for parents at our local schools. We've seen some wonderful changes being made in what the schools offer in their lunch programs and allow in their snacks. Consider becoming an activist in your school district to get changes made that will make a difference in the health of the kids. One night, at a meeting of our local school board, of which I (Dr. Bill) was a member, I raised my hand and said, "I'm concerned about how easy it is for students to get drugs at our school."

The rest of the board members were shocked. "Drugs at our school?"

"Yes, students can get them easily and cheaply," I added.

"What kind of drugs?" they asked.

"Drugs that keep them from learning, cause undesirable behavior, make them aggressive, shorten their attention span, hamper their athletic performance, and even make them fat."

Noticing a bunch of shocked faces, I decided to push harder. "Right now I could walk fifty feet and for a buck get some of these drugs."

That's when they realized I was talking about the junk carbs in the school's vending machines.

Parents and teachers often forget that junk carbs can act like drugs, especially when you partner them with the caffeine, artificial flavors, and chemical colorings found in the soft drinks in school vending machines.

On another occasion I was asked by a group of parents to discuss improving the nutritional content of the food offered in the school's lunch program. I began by asking the principal, "Why do we send our children to school?" He looked at me, rather puzzled. I went on, "In a nutshell, we send our children to school to teach them the tools to succeed in life! What better tool to teach our children than the tools for health? And one of the top tools for health is nutritious eating. Junk food at the school confuses children. Some students conclude that if the school serves it, it must be good for them, even if it's contrary to what they've been taught at home." The principal got the point. You might try this approach with your school principal.

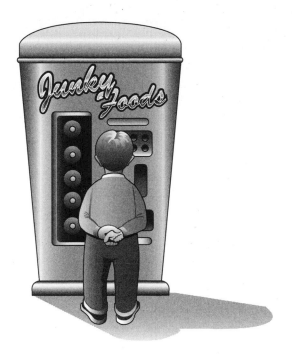

Parents at home (as well as the school health curriculum) teach kids to avoid sugar-sweetened drinks and high-fat, bad-carb foods. Yet these foods are readily available at school. In fact, most school lunch programs offer one bad "kid food" after another, including greasy cheeseburgers, french fries, breaded chicken strips, and sugary juice drinks. Teaching children about "right-track eating" in the lunch room as well as in the classroom is an important addition to the traditional "three R's." As a result of our meeting, a committee of parents and food service personnel was formed to explore nutritious changes in school food offerings. The kindergarten that Dr. Jim's kids went to had a rule regarding bag lunches and snacks: sugar or high-fructose corn syrup could not be one of the first five ingredients.

There are many ways in which you can make a difference. Join the PTA at your children's school, and involve other parents as

SCHOOL LUNCHES TO GROW BIG AND SMART

If you're tired of fighting the junky school lunch program (please don't give up!), here are some suggestions. If the cafeteria menu is available for preview, have your children bring it home and select healthy choices with them. If you prefer to pack your child's lunch, make it so good that she won't be tempted to trade. Here is a list of items to consider putting into your child's lunches. Use creative containers, and mix and match the foods according to your child's age and tastes:

Peanut butter or almond butter sandwich with all-fruit jelly on whole wheat bread

Small servings of fruits or veggies, such as:
- crunchy sliced red, yellow, or green peppers
- cherry tomatoes
- celery sticks filled with cheese spread
- carrot sticks
- raw broccoli florets
- dried apricots
- red grapes
- mixed nuts with dried fruits, such as raisins and cranberries

Container of guacamole dip for the bagged veggies

Avocado slices

6- or 8-ounce container of yogurt

you lobby for healthy school lunches and junk-free vending machines. Parents can influence school policies and cafeteria menus. Many states have passed laws against stocking public school vending machines with sweetened beverages.

Meanwhile, send your child to school with a bag lunch and

String cheese

Awesome Oatmeal-Raisin Cookies (see recipe, page 304)

Homemade muffins with flaxseed meal, raisins, and nuts

Peanut Butter Carob Balls (see recipe, page 305)

8-ounce carton of milk

8-ounce carton of 100 percent juice

Individual favorite fruit (apple, orange, banana, kiwi, peach, etc.)

Veggie-Hummus Wrap (see recipe, page 310)

Peanut Butter Protein Balls (see recipe, page 305)

Mini pizza (see recipe, page 307)

Lettuce roll: large leaf of romaine lettuce filled with sliced turkey, tomato, and low-fat cream cheese, rolled up like a burrito

Whole wheat pita pocket filled with greens, diced veggies, and olive oil–based salad dressing (use really dark greens such as spinach or field greens)

Bean-and-cheese burrito made with a whole wheat tortilla (add tomato or cut-up veggies)

Quesadilla made with a whole wheat tortilla (use low-fat cheese)

Veggie kabob

For more creative school lunch suggestions, visit www.Ask DrSears.com/schoollunches.

---

healthy snacks. Pack foods that you know your child likes so you can be sure he'll eat them and not trade them. (For suggestions for healthy school snacks, see pages 167 and 178.) Remember that the best brain foods are carbs partnered with protein and fiber.

Each day I write a little love note on a Post-it and tape it to her bag of veggies.

◆

My child is into sports, so I attach an action-related note such as "Eat your soccer balls" on the little bag of cherry tomatoes.

GOT MILK?

Many parents I know don't allow their children to drink milk. When I was a kid, adults urged us to drink milk. I'm confused.

As pediatricians we are aware of the different views about milk. Some parents are worried about milk allergies. Others believe that eliminating milk from their child's diet will improve their child's health and behavior in every possible way. It is true that milk is not absolutely necessary for bone health. In 2005 the journal *Pediatrics* published a review article of reputable studies about dairy sources of calcium and bone health and concluded that there was no scientific evidence to support the notion that milk is the preferred source of calcium for bone health. Researchers also found that physical activity during adolescence contributed more to adult bone health than dietary calcium did. (For the best nondairy sources of calcium, see page 268.)

That said, we would rather see kids drink milk than sweetened beverages or even fruit juice. It's true that kids today don't drink as much milk as children did twenty or thirty years ago. Many nutritionists believe the switch from milk to sweetened beverages has contributed to the epidemic of childhood obesity. When kids drink pop or juice instead of milk, they are loading up on empty calories while neglecting an important grow food.

Milk is more than a beverage; it's a nutrient-dense food. An 8-ounce glass of low-fat milk contains 10 grams of protein, healthy carbs, 300 milligrams of calcium, and an ample supply of B vitamins, vitamin D, and minerals. Another nutritional advantage of milk is that it's hard to drink too much of it. Kids can easily guzzle a 24- or 32-ounce sports drink, but milk is much more filling. It's hard to drink more than 8 to 12 ounces, especially with a meal.

Always buy organic milk to minimize your child's exposure to the hormones and antibiotics that are fed to dairy cows. Serve low-fat milk to children over two years of age; children don't need all the fat in whole milk. And consider chocolate milk a yellow-light food — okay for a treat now and then, not daily, and only if it's made with sugar rather than corn syrup.

Milk allergies and intolerance. These two conditions are often confused. Between 3 and 5 percent of children are *allergic* to milk. The usual symptoms of milk allergy are a red, rough, raised rash, especially on the cheeks; respiratory symptoms such as a runny nose, coughing, and wheezing. Allergies to milk are caused by milk protein. Children with mild milk allergies may be able to tolerate yogurt and cheese, since the processing used to make these foods alters the proteins. Children with severe allergies may have to avoid all dairy products.

Milk (lactose) *intolerance* is usually the result of not being able to digest the lactose in milk. Lactose is the carbohydrate in milk, a sugar unique to mammal milk. Infants can digest lactose, but some people lose this ability as they get older, and they experience bloating, abdominal pain, and diarrhea shortly after drinking milk or eating ice cream. Most children who are lactose intolerant can handle a small amount of milk, sipping it slowly rather than guzzling it. Or they can drink lactose-free milk, in which the lactose has already been broken down by added enzymes. Children who are lactose intolerant can usually eat yogurt without any problems, since the culturing process that turns milk into yogurt breaks down some of the lactose. Most lactose-intolerant children can eat cheese, too, especially firm cheeses such as Parmesan, without intestinal upset.

Milk substitutes. Rice milk is not a healthy alternative to cow's milk. It contains mostly carbohydrates, with minimal amounts of protein. Plain soy milk is a more nutritious milk substitute for children who must avoid dairy products. Be aware that flavored soy drinks are made with sugar or corn syrup. Almond "milk" is a nutritious option.

Some parents prefer to give their children goat's milk instead of cow's milk. Goat's milk is less likely to provoke an allergic reaction, because it contains less of the major protein in cow's milk to which some children are allergic, and the protein in goat's milk forms a softer, more digestible curd in the stomach. It also may produce a better "gut feeling" than cow's milk because goat's milk has less lactose, and the fat is easier to digest. There are some nutritional trade-offs when you substitute milk from goats for milk from cows. Goat's milk contains a bit more calcium, vitamin B-6, vitamin A, niacin, potassium, and copper, but cow's milk has much more vitamin B-12 and folic acid. For this reason, if goat's milk is used as a sole source of nutrition (as when used with the proper dilution and supplementation in infant formula), always be sure that the goat's milk you buy is supplemented with folic acid. Also, be sure to buy goat's milk that is certified free of antibiotics and growth hormones (BGH/BST). We recommend Meyenberg goat milk.

HOW MUCH FOOD? HOW MANY CALORIES?

I often wonder how much food our five-year-old should eat. Obesity runs in our family, so I'm concerned about her eating too much. Should I be counting calories for her?

You are wise to be concerned about your child's maintaining a proper weight even at a young age. Chubby kids are likely to become obese adults, and just like adults, children get fat when they take in more calories than they burn up. Yet, in our LEAN Kids

Program, the weight-management program we run in our pediatric practice, we seldom instruct parents to count kids' calories. Besides, calorie-counting diets are likely to fail, because eating is supposed to be a pleasurable thing to do, not a mathematical project.

Children are growing and should be very active. The number of calories they need varies from day to day. Except for very obese children, we don't encourage weight loss in kids. Instead, we help them maintain the same weight for the next year or two. We call this the "no-gain goal." As they grow taller, they automatically "lean out" and achieve their ideal weight.

For most children, it is unnecessary to count calories or measure portion sizes. What is more important is serving them grow foods (see chapter 5). Rather than worrying about how much your daughter eats, turn your attention to what she eats and to how active she is. The fact is, most grow foods are filling without being fattening. Children rarely overeat grow foods.

If you need reassurance that your daughter's appetite is a good match for what her body needs, here's the math:

- Most children from five to twelve years of age who are moderately active need around 30 calories per pound of optimal body weight per day. This works out to between 1,500 and 2,000 calories a day.

- Children burn calories differently from adults. Body types that are lean — "bananas" — burn more calories than chubby, round "apples."

- Activity level affects calorie needs. During strenuous exercise such as running, children can burn an extra 300 calories an hour.

As a general guide, a child weighing 70 pounds needs about 2,000 calories a day, plus 300 to 500 calories depending on her activity level. Here's how those calories look, spread out over a day's meals and snacks:

Breakfast: 500 calories
Midmorning snack: 200 calories
Lunch: 500 calories
Midafternoon snack: 200 calories
Dinner: 500 calories
Before-bed snack: 100 calories

Ideally, these calories are made up of protein, healthy carbs, and healthy fats in the following proportions:

- protein: 15 to 20 percent of total daily calories
- healthy carbs: 50 to 60 percent (depending on activity level)

HOW TO GROW THE HEALTHIEST KID IN THE NEIGHBORHOOD – A REVIEW

The following is a list of the high points of our healthy eating plan. Attach it to your refrigerator as a reminder for your family.

Reminder	Page
☐ Feed your family the *right carbs:* Partner carbs with protein and fiber.	65
☐ Limit sweetened beverages.	76
☐ Limit artificial sweeteners.	85
☐ Survey your kitchen for the "bad words" on food labels.	53, 186
☐ Feed your family the *right fats.*	91
☐ Feed your family more seafood.	98
☐ "Oil" your growing kids; use the best oils.	106
☐ Trim the fat from family foods.	110
☐ Avoid bad fats.	96
☐ Feed your family grow foods.	116

- healthy fats: 25 to 30 percent (mostly from seafood and plant sources)

An appropriate child-size serving of most foods is about the volume of the child's fist. A snack should be one fist size of food. Breakfast, lunch, and dinner may be two to three fist sizes of different foods, although this varies with the hunger and activity level of the child. The stomach stretches during a meal, but you don't want to overstretch it.

Reminder	Page
☐ Teach traffic-light eating.	118
☐ Serve whole grains instead of processed ones.	136
☐ Raise a grazer.	146
☐ Feed your family supersnacks.	163, 167, 178
☐ Exclude excitotoxins from the family's diet.	185
☐ Water your growing kids.	160
☐ Begin the day with a brainy breakfast.	188
☐ Feed your family lots of "phytos."	194
☐ Feed your child immune-boosting foods.	205, 285
☐ Raise a lean family.	210
☐ Enjoy a salad at the beginning of a meal.	282
☐ Teach your child smart food shopping.	237
☐ Buy organic.	259
☐ Be sure your family eats enough omega 3's.	264
☐ Raise veggie lovers.	274
☐ Eat at family-friendly restaurants.	281
☐ Serve healthy school meals.	287

12

Recipes

No matter how nutritious the food you prepare for your children and the strategies you use to serve it, if they don't like the taste, they're unlikely to eat it. Here are some of our favorite recipes that are both healthy and tasty. We have tried to focus these recipes on the twelve superfoods for kids listed on page 55, packaged with or "hidden" in some traditional children's favorites. We have added a few optional special additions to some of the recipes. Use organic sources whenever possible. For more recipes, see our website, www.AskDr.Sears.com/recipes.

SMOOTHIES AND BREAKFASTS

DR. BILL'S SCHOOL-ADE SMOOTHIE
Makes 8 cups

Here's the Sears family recipe that we have been making an average of five days a week for the past eight years. Our whole family enjoys it, as do the families in our pediatric practice who have tried it.

2 cups plain nonfat yogurt
2 cups milk or soy beverage
1 cup frozen blueberries
1 cup mixed frozen fruit:
   strawberries, mango,
   papaya, or pineapple
1 banana
2 tbsp. flaxseeds, ground, or
   flaxseed *oil* for a smoother
   taste
4 ounces tofu
whey protein powder
   (10–12 grams)
1 tbsp. cinnamon
2 tbsp. peanut butter
   (nonhydrogenated)

Special Additions
1–2 servings chocolate-
   or vanilla-flavored
   multivitamin/multimineral
   protein powder
¼ cup raisins (for extra
   sweetness)
2 kiwis (for extra vitamin C)
2 tbsp. wheat germ
1 cup fresh baby spinach
   leaves
1 cup carrot juice
a few ice cubes to chill it for
   better taste

Combine all the ingredients in a blender and blend until smooth. Add more liquid to get the desired consistency. Blend again. Serve immediately, before the air settles and while the mixture has a bubbly milkshake texture.

Besides being tasty and easy to serve, this recipe is nutritionally balanced. Depending on your special additions, it contains around 25 percent protein, 25 percent healthy fats, and 50 percent healthy carbs, in addition to 25 to 30 grams of fiber in 1,200 to 1,400 calories, for 64 ounces.

ASHTON'S SMOOTHIE

Serves 2 kids

While it may sound strange, our granddaughter Ashton loves this recipe. The kale or spinach taste and color are covered up and therefore undetected. This is a great way to get kale (the number-one cancer-fighting vegetable) into your kids.

⅔ cup carrot juice
1 serving vanilla-flavored
   multivitamin/multimineral
   protein powder
⅔ cup frozen blueberries
½ cup uncooked kale or
   spinach

Special Additions
1 tbsp. raisins or ½ frozen
   banana (for extra
   sweetness)

Combine all the ingredients in a blender and blend on high for about one minute.

VEGGIE FRITTATA

Serves about 6

This is a great meal for any time of the day. You can use any combination of veggies. Leftover veggies work great in this dish, and it's an easy way to get a lot of veggies into your child all at once.

2 cups whole-grain bread
   crumbs
2 cups diced uncooked
   spinach
2 cups diced tomatoes
1 cup grated zucchini
1 medium red onion

1 cup sliced mushrooms
2 cups grated Parmesan or
   mozzarella cheese
12 eggs
1 cup milk
garlic salt and pepper to
   taste

Special addition
Garnish with fresh rosemary
   sprigs or mix the chopped
   leaves in before baking.

Preheat the oven to 400°. Grease a 13" x 9" baking dish. Line the dish with bread crumbs, then add the veggies topped with 1 cup of the cheese. In a separate bowl, beat together the eggs, milk, garlic salt, and pepper, and pour the mixture over the cheese. Bake for 25 to 30 minutes. Top with the remaining cheese and bake until the cheese is golden brown.

CHOCOLATE CRÊPES

Makes about 6 12-inch crêpes

This is a special festive meal that our family enjoys. Everyone can put their own favorite topping on them.

8 egg whites
1 serving chocolate-flavored
   multivitamin/multimineral
   protein powder

1 cup old-fashioned (regular)
   oatmeal
½ cup low-fat cottage cheese
dash of salt

Combine all of the ingredients in a blender and blend until smooth. Heat a medium-size skillet over medium heat. Coat the skillet with olive oil or cooking spray (nonhydrogenated). Pour the batter (it will be runny) into the skillet to make thin crêpes. Let crêpes cook for about 30 seconds on each side. Top with favorite toppings, such as fresh berries or other fruit, nut butter, yogurt, honey, cinnamon, or a bit of whipped cream.

AWESOME OATMEAL

Cook a family-size portion of steel-cut oatmeal in a Crock-Pot overnight. Your family will awaken to a breakfast of hot oatmeal. Put a dollop of yogurt and a serving of blueberries on top. Sprinkle on some cinnamon. Enjoy!

SNACKS

DR. BILL'S TERRIFIC TRAIL MIX

Makes 2½ cups; 1 serving = 1 palmful

Caution: Nuts and seeds pose a choking hazard to children under three or four years of age.

½ cup raw walnuts	*Special Additions*
⅓ cup raw pecans	other nuts your child prefers
⅓ cup raw pistachio nut meats	soy nuts
¼ cup raw sunflower seeds	unsweetened carob chips
⅓ cup raw pumpkin seeds	a few semisweet chocolate
⅓ cup raisins	chips
⅓ cup dried cranberries or	
cherries	

Combine all of the ingredients in a bowl. Encourage your child to scoop each of these ingredients out of the package and toss them together in the bowl.

HEARTY HUMMUS

This is a very easy dip to whip together. Hummus makes raw veggies more appealing.

2 15-ounce cans of chickpeas,
   not drained
3 cloves garlic
¼ cup tahini (sesame seed
   butter)
1 tbsp. extra-virgin olive oil
¼ cup lemon juice

3 tbsp. water
¼ tsp. salt

Special additions
cilantro
red bell pepper
sun-dried tomatoes

Drain the chickpeas, reserving ¼ cup of the liquid. In a food processor, mince the garlic, then add the rest of the ingredients, plus the chickpea liquid. Process for about 3 minutes or until smooth. Serve with raw vegetables or whole wheat pita triangles. Refrigerate any unused portion.

CHOCOLATE OATMEAL FLAX COOKIES

Makes 3 to 4 dozen

1 cup softened butter, canola
   oil, or other
   nonhydrogenated oil
   spread
1 cup honey (or to taste)
½ cup pure maple syrup or
   ½ cup xylitol
2 eggs
1½ tsp. vanilla
1¼ cups whole-wheat pastry
   flour
½ cup flaxseed meal

2 tsp. baking soda
1 tsp. salt
1 tbsp. cinnamon
1 tsp. nutmeg
1½–2 cups oats
12 ounces dark chocolate or
   carob chips

Special Additions
2 tbsp. brewer's yeast
favorite nuts or seeds

(*continued on next page*)

Mix the butter, honey, maple syrup, eggs, and vanilla together. In a separate bowl, combine the remaining ingredients, except the oats and chocolate chips. Stir the dry ingredients into the wet. Add the oats and chocolate chips. Refrigerate the dough until it is firm. Roll teaspoonfuls of dough into balls and place them on an ungreased cookie sheet. Bake at 350° for about 10 minutes (less for chewy cookies, more for crispy ones).

AWESOME OATMEAL-RAISIN COOKIES

Makes 3 to 4 dozen

Instead of using maple syrup or honey, try sweetening the cookies with xylitol or date sugar.

½ cup pure maple syrup or honey
½ cup grapeseed oil, canola oil, or butter
½ tsp. baking soda
1 tbsp. ground cinnamon
1 tsp. vanilla
¼ tsp. baking powder
¼ tsp. sea salt
1 egg
1½ cups oats or granola

1 cup whole wheat pastry flour, or ⅓ cup almond meal and ⅔ cup flour
1 cup raisins

Special Additions
½ cup chopped walnuts
8 ounces silken-soft tofu instead of oil
½ cup carob chips

Heat oven to 375°. Combine all the ingredients except the oats, flour, and raisins and mix thoroughly. Stir in the oats, flour, and raisins. Drop the batter by teaspoonfuls on a cookie sheet and bake until light brown.

PEANUT BUTTER CAROB BALLS

Makes 30 small balls

Warning: Don't put the whole batch on the table in front of your family. These cookies are so tasty that you'll have a hard time limiting yourself to one or two at a time. We love them! (Refrigerated balls stored in an airtight container keep for up to a month.)

½ cup carob powder
½ cup honey
½ cup crunchy peanut butter
    (nonhydrogenated)
½ cup raw sunflower seeds

½ cup sesame seeds
½ cup oats or quinoa flakes

Special Addition
¼ to ½ cup flaxseed meal

Mix all of the ingredients together by hand. Form the batter into bite-size balls and roll them in shredded coconut.

PEANUT BUTTER PROTEIN BALLS

Makes 3 dozen

Our kids love these, and so do we. They are a healthy snack as well as a dessert. Kids like to help roll them into balls or other fun shapes.

½ cup honey (or less, to taste)
⅔ cup natural peanut butter
    (nonhydrogenated)
1 cup chocolate-flavored
    multivitamin/multimineral
    protein powder
3½ cups crispy rice cereal

Special Addition
diced raisins or dates

(continued on next page)

Mix the honey, peanut butter, and protein powder together completely (this is easier if the honey and peanut butter are room temperature). Slowly add the rice cereal and carefully stir until mixed. Use a cookie baller or your hands to roll the mixture into balls of desired size. Refrigerate the balls for about 30 minutes to firm them up.

LUNCHES OR DINNERS

MARTHA'S LUSCIOUS LENTIL SOUP

Serves 4 to 5

1½ cups washed lentils
3 tbsp. butter
3 garlic cloves, minced
2 small onions, finely chopped
1 large stalk celery, chopped
¼ cup celery leaves, chopped
3–4 carrots, thickly sliced
⅓ cup raw brown rice
2 tbsp. fresh parsley or
 cilantro, chopped

1 tsp. salt
All-purpose natural seasoning,
 to taste
Black pepper, freshly ground,
 to taste

Special Additions
2 cups shredded spinach
grated Parmesan cheese

Place lentils in a bowl and cover with cold water. Let them soak while you prepare the other vegetables. Heat the butter in a large pot. Add the garlic, onions, celery, and celery leaves, and cook while stirring for 5 minutes over medium heat or until the onions have wilted. Add the carrots, rice, parsley, and lentils. Add 1½ quarts of water and seasonings.

Bring the soup to a boil. Cover it and simmer until the lentils, rice, and vegetables are tender (around 1½ hours). If you are including the special additions, add the spinach 20 minutes before serving. Garnish with the Parmesan cheese just before serving.

PRETTY PIZZA

This recipe is a hit in our home. The children love to make their own pizzas. They can use the toppings to make fun designs, faces, or words. Allow grated carrots or zucchini to be hair, sliced tomatoes to be ears, sliced olives to be eyes, an upside-down slice of mushroom to be a nose, and a red bell pepper slice to be a mouth. We have used this as a party activity and a meal. Diced veggies can easily be hidden in the sauce as well.

whole wheat tortillas
marinara sauce or pizza sauce
low-fat mozzarella cheese,
   grated
chopped veggies

Special Additions
chicken chunks
tofu cubes
sliced olives

Preheat the oven to 425°. Place each tortilla on a baking sheet or piece of foil. Spread with marinara or pizza sauce. Sprinkle cheese over the sauce and add your favorite veggie toppings. Place in the oven and cook until the cheese starts to turn golden brown. Allow to cool for at least one minute before serving.

DR. BILL'S SUPER SALAD

Serves 2

2 cups baby spinach
1 cup arugula
1 cup chopped or wedged
    tomatoes or cherry
    tomatoes
2 tsp. turmeric
¼ cup walnut halves
¼ cup sunflower seeds
¼ cup raisins
sprinkle of lemon or lime juice
10 Greek olives, sliced
2 tbsp. olive oil

Special Additions
2 tbsp. hummus
cranberries, dried
pine nuts
blueberries
¼ cup square tofu chunks, firm
sprinkle of Parmesan cheese
grilled wild salmon fillet on
    top

Combine all of the ingredients in a large bowl and toss.

MEATLOAF MUFFINS

Serves 6 to 8

This is a fun version of traditional meat loaf. Kids love having a couple muffins that they can eat with their hands. The veggies in this dish become invisible after it is cooked. Leftover muffins become great snacks.

2 pounds ground turkey or
    chicken
2 eggs
1 cup whole-grain bread
    crumbs (preferably dried)
1½ cups fresh spinach, diced
2 plum tomatoes, diced

4 cloves garlic, chopped
1 red onion, diced
¼ cup Worcestershire sauce
1½ cups grated low-fat
    Monterey Jack cheese

Special Additions
¼ cup honey (or less, to
   taste) — it gives a
   delightfully sweet taste

hot pepper sauce to taste

Preheat the oven to 350°. In a large bowl, mix all ingredients until completely combined. Spoon the mixture into a lightly greased muffin tin (any extra can go into a small loaf pan) and bake for 50 to 60 minutes or until the meatloaf is firm to the touch. Remove from the tin and serve.

SALMON LETTUCE TACOS

Serves 5 to 8

This is a fun, unconventional way to serve salmon. You can use corn tortillas for the shell if the lettuce shell does not go over well.

1 pound of Alaskan salmon
   fillets
5–8 large leaves of Romaine
   lettuce used as shells (or
   other large-leaf green
   lettuce)
1 tbsp. olive oil
1 avocado, sliced
1 tomato, diced

½ red onion, sliced
cilantro
full-fat plain yogurt or sour
   half-and-half
salsa

Special Additions
other favorite taco toppings

Slice the salmon fillets into 1-inch strips. Sauté in olive oil in a large skillet until fully cooked (about 5 minutes). Place the remaining ingredients in separate bowls and set them on the table or buffet area. Let everyone prepare their own taco (if age appropriate). Place a couple slices of salmon into the lettuce shell and then add the toppings.

PRETTY PASTA SHELLS

Serves 6 to 8

This nutritious spin on a classic Italian dish is one of our family's favorites. The optional tofu is great for extra protein and makes it a more complete meal. The tofu melts in with the ricotta cheese, so you can't even tell it is there.

1 pound large pasta shells or manicotti tubes

16 ounces frozen spinach, thawed and drained

1 15-ounce container of low-fat ricotta

1 cup grated Parmesan cheese

1 tbsp. fennel seeds (or less, to taste)

1 tsp. basil

30 ounces organic marinara sauce

1½ cups grated low-fat mozzarella cheese

Special Addition

8 ounces firm tofu, chopped

Preheat the oven to 375°. Cook the pasta according to the directions on the package. Mix the spinach, ricotta, Parmesan cheese, fennel seeds, and basil in a bowl. Cover the bottom of a large casserole dish with a 1-inch layer of marinara sauce. Carefully spoon the spinach/cheese mixture into the cooked pasta shells and place them in rows in the casserole dish. Cover with the desired amount of marinara sauce and bake for about 30 minutes. Cover with mozzarella cheese and bake an additional 10 minutes.

VEGGIE-HUMMUS WRAP

Makes 2

This is a great mini-meal or on-the-go snack. It is a good meal for children to help prepare.

2 whole wheat tortillas or
   whole wheat pita bread
½ cup hummus (any flavor)
1 cup diced veggies of your
   choice

Special Additions
avocado slices
grated low-fat cheese

Spread hummus evenly over each tortilla. Sprinkle veggies on top. Roll up the tortilla and serve.

TURKEY-VEGGIE SALAD SANDWICH

Makes 1 large sandwich

This simple yet tasty meal on the go is a great use of leftovers. It's a good way to get out of an "ordinary sandwich" rut.

3–4 ounces chopped cooked
   turkey or chicken
1 tbsp. plain low-fat yogurt
1 tbsp. mayonnaise (or canola
   oil low-fat mayonnaise)
½ cup diced raw veggies of
   your choice (you can use an
   electric chopper or food
   processor)

¼ cups raisins
2 slices whole-grain bread or
   pita, plain or toasted

Special Addition
curry powder to taste

Combine the chicken or turkey with the yogurt and mayonnaise (and curry powder, if desired) in a small bowl. Then add the veggies and raisins. Spoon the mixture onto the bread.

TURKEY PIE

Serves 6 to 8

You can include other vegetables, too, or use soy cheese and a soy meat substitute instead. Toddlers love to feed this to themselves.

6 medium-size yams or sweet
   potatoes, chopped (keep
   skins on) and mashed
2 pounds lean ground turkey
   or chicken, browned
2 cups corn, fresh, frozen, or
   canned
2 cups green beans (raw is
   best)

1 cup tomato, diced
2 cups low-fat cheddar cheese
1 cup low-fat Monterey Jack
   cheese
1 can kidney beans
salt and pepper to taste

Preheat the oven to 350°. Steam the chopped yams or sweet potatoes until tender. Transfer them to a bowl and beat until creamy. Layer ingredients into a large casserole dish as follows, adding salt and pepper to taste every few layers: half the mashed potatoes, turkey, corn, beans, tomatoes, cheddar cheese, remainder of mashed potatoes, and Monterey Jack cheese. Bake for about 30 minutes.

CHEESY PIE

Serves 6 to 8

This is a Sears family favorite. It is packed with veggies, protein, and calcium. It is a great one-dish meal.

1 pound lean ground turkey,
   chicken, or soy meat
   substitute

3 medium zucchini, chopped
3 green onions, chopped
1 tsp. basil

1 tsp. Italian seasoning
4 organic free-range eggs
⅓ cup nonfat milk or soy milk
4 ounces low-fat cream cheese, cubed (it is easier to cut if frozen)

½ cup low-fat mozzarella cheese, grated
½ cup low-fat cheddar cheese, grated
salt to taste

Preheat the oven to 425°. Brown your choice of meat or meat substitute in a skillet. Cover the bottom of a large pie pan with the meat. Layer on the zucchini and green onions. Add the basil and Italian seasoning (and salt, if desired). Whisk the eggs and milk together and pour into the pie pan. Sprinkle all three cheeses on top. Bake for 30 minutes.

PENNE WITH SALMON AND PEAS*

Serves 6 to 8

Kids love peas, cheesy sauces, and little tubes of penne pasta, so most will like this mild recipe. The proportions provided here will feed a big family or leave time-pressed parents with great leftovers.

1 tsp. salt
4 cups penne pasta
2 cups frozen peas
3 tbsp. butter (preferably unsalted)
3 tbsp. all-purpose flour
1½ to 2 cups warm milk (whole or 2 percent)

¼ cup shredded mozzarella
1½ to 2 cups crumbled wild salmon, slightly cooked
Freshly grated Parmesan cheese

(continued on next page)

* Thanks, Randy and Carla, at VitalChoice Seafood Co. (www.VitalChoice.com), for the recipes for salmon and seafood marinade.

Preheat the oven to 350°. Bring a large saucepan three-quarters full of water to a boil, and add salt and penne. Stir well and cook 9 to 10 minutes or according to instructions on package. (Do not cook until soft, as it will cook further in the oven.) In the final 3 minutes of cooking, add the frozen peas. Drain and transfer to a large, deep bowl. Meanwhile, in a saucepan, melt butter over low heat. With a wire whisk, briskly stir in the flour until mixed (about 1 minute). Gradually pour in the warm milk, stirring until smooth. Stir in the cheese and add additional milk if necessary. Toss the pasta and peas with the cheese sauce. Gently fold in the salmon. Spread the mixture into a lightly greased baking dish and sprinkle with Parmesan cheese. Cover and bake for twenty minutes. Allow it to cool for five minutes, and serve.

To create a more adult-oriented version that older kids may also enjoy, see the Adult Variation, below.

Adult Variation
Replace ¼ cup of mozzarella with ¼ cup goat cheese, crumbled. Reconstitute 2 ounces of sun-dried tomatoes in boiling hot water, slice, and add to cheese sauce along with the salmon. Stir in these four herbs after stirring in the cheese(s): ½ tsp. dried (or 1 tsp. fresh) oregano; ½ tsp. dried (or 1 tsp. fresh) thyme; ½ tsp. dried (or 1 tsp. fresh) basil; and 1 tsp. dried (or 1 tbsp. fresh) parsley.

SALMON WITH SAVORY MARINADE

Serves 4

¼ cup olive oil
1 tbsp. lemon pepper
  seasoning
1 tbsp. fresh-squeezed lemon
  juice

1–2 tsp. dill weed
1–2 tsp. fennel seeds
1–2 tsp. soy sauce
Four 6-ounce salmon fillets

Special Additions
crushed garlic
grated fresh ginger
brown sugar

In a large bowl, combine all ingredients except the salmon and mix well. An hour or so before cooking, cut the fillets into individual portions and completely coat them with well-stirred marinade. (Tip: Place the marinade and fish pieces in a large Ziploc bag, close carefully, and turn until all pieces are evenly coated. Place in the refrigerator until needed.)

Preheat the grill or broiler to high. Place the fish on the grill or under the broiler, skin side down. The fish will cook quickly, so be attentive. (Remember the "ten minutes per inch" rule.) Start the thinner pieces after thicker ones. The fish is done when the meat flakes apart and is opaque all the way through.

FANTASTIC FISH STICKS

Cut salmon, tuna, or halibut into strips about the size of your pinky. Place the pieces of fish in the savory seafood marinade (see above). Have your child help. Call them "fish in a bag." Let the fish marinate in the refrigerator for at least one hour. Place marinated strips on a baking rack under a broiler for around five minutes. Don't overcook! The fish is done when it flakes easily with a fork.

HAPPY HALIBUT

Serves 4

2 cups Dijon mustard
2 tbsp. crushed fresh garlic
1 tbsp. lemon pepper
2 tsp. fines herbes seasoning
   (or a combination of
   parsley, chervil, chives,
   tarragon, and coriander)
½ cup white or red wine
   vinegar, or a mixture of half
   fresh lemon juice and half
   vinegar

¼ cup extra-virgin olive oil
⅓ cup light soy sauce
Four 6-ounce halibut steaks

Special Additions
3–4 shakes hot sauce
red pepper flakes to taste

In a bowl or blender whisk together the mustard, garlic, lemon pepper, and fines herbes. Add the vinegar, olive oil, soy sauce, and any optional flavorings, if desired. Place the steaks in the marinade for 1 hour covered at room temperature. Broil or grill the steaks for four minutes on one side and approximately six minutes on the other.

DESSERTS

CREATIVE POPSICLES

Once they've tasted these popsicles, your children will forget about the store-bought kind. These recipes also work for smoothies (more liquid may need to be added).

Chocolate Raspberry

1 cup soy milk, plain or chocolate, or low-fat milk

¼ cup chocolate-flavored multivitamin/multimineral protein powder

½ cup organic red raspberries, frozen

2 tbsp. flaxseed meal

Strawberries and Crème

1 cup soy milk, plain or vanilla, or low-fat milk

¼ cup vanilla-flavored multivitamin/multimineral protein powder

½ cup strawberries, frozen or fresh

dribble of honey

2 tbsp. flaxseed meal

Chocolate Banana Peanut Butter

1 cup soy milk, plain or chocolate, or low-fat milk

¼ cup chocolate-flavored multivitamin/multimineral protein powder

2 tbsp. peanut butter (nonhydrogenated)

1 banana, fresh or frozen

2 tbsp. flaxseed meal

(continued on next page)

Orangesicle

1 cup soy milk, plain or vanilla, or low-fat milk

¼ cup vanilla-flavored multivitamin/multimineral protein powder

2 tbsp. frozen orange juice concentrate

1 tsp. vanilla extract

2 tbsp. flaxseed meal

Combine all the ingredients in a blender and blend on high for 1 minute or until smooth. Pour the mixture into Popsicle molds or small cups with sticks in them. Freeze and enjoy!

Special Additions

Add vegetables to the mix for added nutrition. If you do it carefully, they will be undetected. Use veggies that will be camouflaged by the color of the Popsicle. For example, use carrots in the Orangesicle; red bell pepper in the Strawberries and Crème, and kale in the Chocolate Banana Peanut Butter.

GUILT-FREE SOFT-SERVE "ICE CREAM"

2 frozen bananas, cut up
splash of milk or soy milk

Remove frozen bananas from the freezer and allow them to thaw for two minutes. Put them in a food processor and process into a nice thick cream. Scoop into a cup and serve.

Special Additions

frozen berries or other fruit

vanilla extract

kale

spinach

You can process any of these additional ingredients into the bananas to make different flavors of "ice cream." The kale or fresh spinach makes it a nice green color, and the taste of the veggie can't be detected.

DR. BILL'S QUICK GELATO

Place a 6- to 8-ounce container of your favorite fruit and yogurt mixture in the freezer for 45 minutes. Presto, you have a quick gelato-like dessert.

Special Additions
almonds
fruit toppings

Index

About the Authors

William Sears, M.D., and Martha Sears, R.N., are the pediatric experts to whom American parents are increasingly turning for advice and information on all aspects of pregnancy, birth, childcare, and family nutrition. Dr. Sears received his pediatric training at Harvard Medical School's Children's Hospital and Toronto's Hospital for Sick Children. He has practiced as a pediatrician for more than thirty years and is associate clinical professor of pediatrics at the University of California School of Medicine, Irvine. Martha Sears is a registered nurse, childbirth educator, and breastfeeding consultant. Their many bestselling books include the twelve previous parenting guides in the Sears Parenting Library. The Searses are the parents of eight children. Their sons, Drs. Robert and James Sears, are both board-certified pediatricians at the Sears Family Pediatric Practice in San Clemente, California. All four authors live in southern California.

Look for these other books
in the Sears Parenting Library

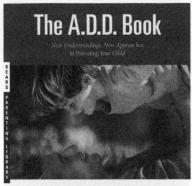

Effective strategies that reach beyond drug therapies to improve cognitive abilities, reduce hyperactivity, and help children with A.D.D. flourish

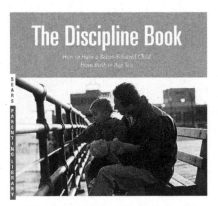

Everything you need to know about managing and preventing behavior problems in your child so that good conduct comes naturally

The bestselling parenting guides for a new generation
Available in paperback wherever books are sold

Look for these other books
in the Sears Parenting Library

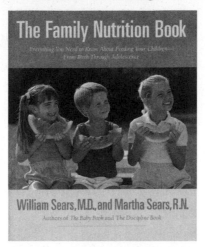

The basics of healthy eating — including a crash course in the six essential nutrient groups required for optimal health: fats, carbohydrates, proteins, vitamins, minerals, and fiber

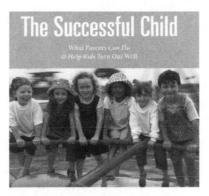

Practical information and examples you can use to help your child become healthy, happy, well-adjusted, and morally grounded

The bestselling parenting guides for a new generation
Available in paperback wherever books are sold

LITTLE, BROWN AND COMPANY

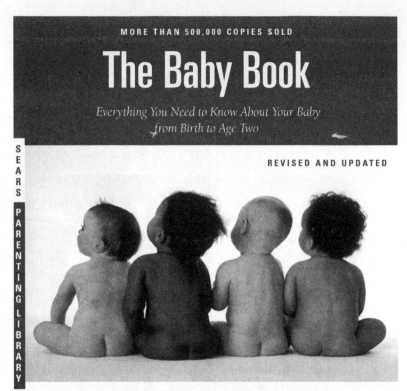